Patient Perspectives in Pulmonary Surgery

Editor

ALESSANDRO BRUNELLI

THORACIC SURGERY CLINICS

www.thoracic.theclinics.com

Consulting Editor

MARK K. FERGUSON

November 2012 • Volume 22 • Number 4

ELSEVIER

1600 John F. Kennedy Boulevard • Suite 1800 • Philadelphia, Pennsylvania 19103-2899

http://www.theclinics.com

THORACIC SURGERY CLINICS Volume 22, Number 4
November 2012 ISSN 1547-4127, ISBN-13: 978-1-4557-4896-9

Editor: Barbara Cohen-Kligerman
Developmental Editor: Teia Stone

Thoracic Surgery Clinics (ISSN 1547-4127) is published quarterly by Elsevier Inc., 360 Park Avenue South, New York, NY 10010-1710. Months of publication are February, May, August, and November. Business and editorial offices: 1600 John F. Kennedy Boulevard, Suite 1800, Philadelphia, PA 19103-2899. Periodicals postage paid at New York, NY, and additional mailing offices. Subscription prices are $335.00 per year (US individuals), $433.00 per year (US institutions), $159.00 per year (US Students), $416.00 per year (Canadian individuals), $547.00 per year (Canadian institutions), $216.00 per year (Canadian and foreign students), $443.00 per year (foreign individuals), and $547.00 per year (foreign institutions). Foreign air speed delivery is included in all Clinics' subscription prices. All prices are subject to change without notice. **POSTMASTER: Send address changes to Thoracic Surgery Clinics, Elsevier Health Sciences Division, Subscription Customer Service, 3251 Riverport Lane, Maryland Heights, MO 63043. Customer Service (orders, claims, online, change of address): Telephone: 1-800-654-2452 (U.S. and Canada); 314-447-8871 (outside U.S. and Canada). Fax: 314-447-8029. Email: journalscustomerservice-usa@elsevier.com (for print support); journalsonlinesupport-usa@elsevier.com (for online support).**

Reprints. For copies of 100 or more, of articles in this publication, please contact Commercial Rights Department, Elsevier Inc., 360 Park Avenue South, New York, NY 10010-1710. Tel: (212) 633-3812; Fax: (212) 462-1935; E-mail: reprints@elsevier.com.

Thoracic Surgery Clinics is covered in *MEDLINE/PubMed (Index Medicus)* and *EMBASE/Excerpta Medica.*

Printed and bound by CPI Group (UK) Ltd, Croydon, CR0 4YY

Transferred to digital print 2012

Contributors

CONSULTING EDITOR

MARK K. FERGUSON, MD
Professor of Surgery, Section of Cardiac and
Thoracic Surgery, The University of Chicago
Medical Center, Chicago, Illinois

GUEST EDITOR

ALESSANDRO BRUNELLI, MD
Chief, Section of Minimally Invasive Thoracic
Surgery, Vice-Director, Division of Thoracic
Surgery, Ospedali Riuniti Ancona, Ancona, Italy

AUTHORS

J. HERMAN BLAKE, PhD
Office of the Vice President for Academic
Affairs and Provost, Humanities Scholar in
Resident, Medical University of South Carolina,
Charleston, South Carolina

ALESSANDRO BRUNELLI, MD
Chief, Section of Minimally Invasive Thoracic
Surgery, Vice-Director, Division of Thoracic
Surgery, Ospedali Riuniti Ancona, Ancona, Italy

ANNETTE J. DeVITO DABBS, PhD, RN
Department of Acute & Tertiary Care, School of
Nursing, University of Pittsburgh, Pittsburgh,
Pennsylvania

MARY AMANDA DEW, PhD
Departments of Psychiatry, Psychology,
Epidemiology and Biostatistics, University of
Pittsburgh, Pittsburgh, Pennsylvania

ANDREA F. DiMARTINI, MD
Departments of Psychiatry and Surgery,
School of Medicine, University of Pittsburgh;
Starzl Transplant Institute, University of
Pittsburgh Medical Center, Pittsburgh,
Pennsylvania

DOMINIC EMERSON, MD
Division of Thoracic Surgery, Department of
Surgery, Georgetown University Medical
Center, Washington, DC

MARK K. FERGUSON, MD
Professor of Surgery, Section of Cardiac and
Thoracic Surgery, The University of Chicago
Medical Center, Chicago, Illinois

D. FITZSIMMONS, PhD
Swansea Centre for Health Economics,
Swansea University, Swansea, United
Kingdom

SABHA GANAI, MD, PhD
Surgical Oncology Fellow, Department of
Surgery, The University of Chicago Medical
Center, Chicago, Illinois

JOHN R. HANDY Jr, MD, HonD
Director, Providence Thoracic Surgery
Program; Co-Director, Providence Thoracic
Oncology Program, Providence Cancer
Center, Portland, Oregon

JIMMIE HOLLAND, MD
Memorial Sloan-Kettering Cancer Center,
New York

C.D. JOHNSON, MChir, FRCS
University Surgical Unit, University of
Southampton School of Medicine,
Southampton University Hospital,
Southampton, United Kingdom

**CHRISTINA JONES, BSc, MPhil, PhD, CSci,
MBACP, DipH**
Nurse Consultant in Critical Care
Rehabilitation, Whiston Hospital, Prescot,
United Kingdom; Honorary Reader,
Department of Musculoskeletal Biology,
Institute of Aging and Chronic Disease,
University of Liverpool, Liverpool,
United Kingdom

MICHAEL KOLLER, PhD
Center for Clinical Studies, University Hospital
Regensburg, Regensburg, Germany

**ERIC LIM, MB ChB, MD, MSc (Biostatistics),
FRCS (C-Th)**
Consultant Thoracic Surgeon, Imperial
College and The Academic Division of
Thoracic Surgery, The Royal Brompton
Hospital; Consultant Thoracic Surgeon,
Imperial College, London, United Kingdom

M. BLAIR MARSHALL, MD
Associate Professor of Surgery, Georgetown
University School of Medicine; Chief, Division
of Thoracic Surgery, Department of Surgery,
Georgetown University Medical Center,
Washington, DC

CECILIA POMPILI, MD
Division of Thoracic Surgery, Ospedali Riuniti
Ancona, Ancona, Italy

GAETANO ROCCO, MD, FRCSEd
Director, Department of Thoracic Surgery and
Oncology; Chief, Division of Thoracic Surgery,
National Cancer Institute, Pascale Foundation,
Naples, Italy

EMILY M. ROSENBERGER, BA
Department of Clinical and Translational
Science, School of Medicine, University of
Pittsburgh, Pittsburgh, Pennsylvania

ROBERT M. SADE, MD
Professor of Surgery, Director, Department of
Surgery, Institute of Human Values in Health
Care, Medical University of South Carolina,
Charleston, South Carolina

MARY KAY SCHWEMMER, JD
Adjunct Professor of Law, Charleston School of
Law, Charleston, South Carolina

ARIELLE M. SCHWERD, BA
Memorial Sloan-Kettering Cancer Center,
New York

MARK WEINBERGER, PhD, MPH
IMA Clinical Research, Tarrytown, New York

TALIA WEISS, MA
Clinical Psychology, Health Emphasis Ferkauf
Graduate School of Psychology, Yeshiva
University and Memorial Sloan-Kettering
Cancer Center, New York

S. WHEELWRIGHT, MA
University Surgical Unit, University of
Southampton School of Medicine,
Southampton University Hospital,
Southampton, United Kingdom

ROGER D. YUSEN, MD, MPH
Division of Pulmonary and Critical Care
Medicine, Washington University School of
Medicine, St Louis, Missouri

Contents

Psychological responses to lung cancer have changed over the past 30 years as perceptions of the disease have changed. Previously seen as a fatal diagnosis, it is now regarded as a cancer whose treatment is increasingly effective as the science of the disease advances. The stigma of smoking is diminishing as more is learned about genetic factors and as more nonsmokers are diagnosed. Support groups are now widely available. The increasing social support and greater knowledge of lung cancer provide a more supportive environment in which patients cope with lung cancer today compared with 30 years ago.

There is mounting recognition that, to aid surgical decision making, treatment efficacy needs to be measured in a variety of ways, with health-related quality of life now widely regarded as an important outcome in pulmonary surgical populations. The aim of this review is to provide a comprehensive overview of the key issues to consider if an investigator wishes to incorporate health-related quality of life assessment into trials and studies of pulmonary surgery, drawing on recent studies of lung cancer surgery as an example.

This article assesses the impact of pulmonary resection on quality of life by means of a systematic quantitative review of the available literature. Perioperative changes in quality of life scales were measured by the Cohen's effect size method (mean change of the variable divided by its baseline standard deviation). After lobectomy, most quality-of-life scales differed slightly from preoperative values but tended to recover from the first evaluation time point up to 12 months after surgery. After pneumonectomy, most scales showed a stable or declining trend from the first evaluation up to 12 months after surgery.

Quality of life (QOL) after medical interventions is paramount to the patient considering treatment recommendations. To understand QOL in thoracic surgery patients, one must examine the outcomes patients prioritize (preferences) from successful surgical therapy, overall functional status of thoracic surgery patients, the literature addressing QOL after thoracic surgery (TS) and the possible benefit of minimally invasive TS, and, finally, future directions of TS postoperative QOL research. The primary focus of this article is lung cancer surgery with mention of other thoracic disease such as empyema, pneumothorax, or emphysema, as well.

Examination of the preferences of patients with lung cancer suggests that the ideal therapy may not be based on standard outcome measures such as survival, but should also consider the morbidity, adverse effects, and convenience of the treatment. Functional outcomes after lung resection have particular importance in guiding decision making in high-risk operative candidates. In this article, quality-of-life measures are reviewed in the context of guiding choices between operative and nonoperative therapies in a shared decision-making model for high-risk candidates for lung resection.

Patients recovering from critical illness may suffer from physical, psychological, and cognitive problems that have a negative impact on their health-related quality of life. To ensure that patients return as close as possible to their previous physical and mental health, their rehabilitation needs should be assessed and an appropriate program started. Both early mobilization and physical rehabilitation while the patient is still in the intensive care unit and manualized rehabilitation after discharge are beneficial. It is important to assess the rehabilitation needs of patients and target physiotherapy and counseling resources at those patients with the greatest need.

Although lung transplantation is an accepted treatment for many individuals with severe lung disease, transplant candidates and recipients experience a range of psychosocial stressors that begin at the initiation of the transplant evaluation and continue throughout patients' wait for donor lungs, their perioperative recovery, and their long-term adjustment to posttransplant life. Transplant programs should strive to incorporate evidence-based interventions that aim to improve physical functioning, psychological distress, global quality of life, and medical adherence as well as to integrate symptom management and palliative care strategies throughout the pre- and posttransplantation course.

From Laennec's invention of the stethoscope in 1816 to the recently introduced Sapien transcatheter aortic valve replacement, the increasing complexity of health care technology has altered the relationship between patients and physicians, usually for the better. Telemedicine, the provision of medical services through electronic media, has dramatically changed how the patient and physician interact and how medical care is delivered. Many studies of physicians' perceptions of electronic communication with patients have documented recognition of benefits as well as a consistent chorus of concerns about confidentiality, increased workload, inappropriate use, and medicolegal issues.

Barriers can arise if surgeons are unable to effectively convey information on benefits and risks or are unwilling to offer management choices based on patients' preferences. Facilitating shared decision making, allowing patients to carefully think and consider the alternatives, and empowering them to share in the decision-making process improve patient satisfaction and treatment adherence and represent the hallmark of an excellent clinician.

Patient safety has been the subject of surgical investigation for the past century. A specific focus on safety and medical errors has incited public attention, government oversight, and research funding. Traditional efforts have been focused on the individual responsible for the "mistake," while current procedure focuses on a systems approach. A critical analysis of medical errors, their frequency and cause, and outcomes associated with their occurrence has allowed the identification of system-based issues and the implementation of corrective changes to improve these systems. Constant vigilance examining errors and how they occur will allow identification of strategies to reduce errors.

Clinical and nonclinical indicators of performance are meant to provide the surgeon with tools to identify weaknesses to be improved. The World Health Organization's Performance Evaluation Systems represent a multidimensional approach to quality measurement based on several categories made of different indicators. Indicators for patient satisfaction may include overall perceived quality, accessibility, humanization and patient involvement, communication, and trust in health care providers. Patient satisfaction is included among nonclinical indicators of performance in thoracic surgery and is increasingly recognized as one of the outcome measures for delivered quality of care.

THORACIC SURGERY CLINICS

FORTHCOMING ISSUES

February 2013
Management of Benign and Malignant Pleural Effusions
Cliff Choong, MBBS, *Guest Editor*

May 2013
Lung Cancer, Part I: Screening, Diagnosis and Staging
Jean Deslauriers, MD, F.G. Pearson, MD, and Farid M. Shamji MBBS (UK), *Guest Editors*

June 2013
Lung Cancer, Part II: Surgery and Adjuvant Therapy
Jean Deslauriers, MD, F.G. Pearson, MD, and Farid M. Shamji MBBS (UK), *Guest Editors*

RECENT ISSUES

August 2012
Surgical Management of Infectious Pleuropulmonary Diseases
Gaetano Rocco, MD, *Guest Editor*

May 2012
The Lymphatic System in Thoracic Oncology
Federico Venuta, MD, and Erino A. Rendina, MD, *Guest Editors*

February 2012
Current Management Guidelines in Thoracic Surgery
M. Blair Marshall, MD, *Guest Editor*

RELATED INTEREST

Surgical Clinics of North America Volume 92, Issue 4 (August 2012)
Recent Advances and Future Directions in Trauma Care
LtCOL Jeremy W. Cannon, MD, SM, *Guest Editor*
Available at http://www.surgical.theclinics.com/

NOW AVAILABLE FOR YOUR iPhone and iPad

Preface
Patient Perspectives in Pulmonary Surgery

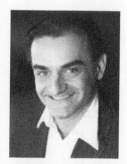

Alessandro Brunelli, MD
Guest Editor

In the modern health care system, patient-centered outcomes have become an important aspect of the evaluation and selection of the most appropriate treatment. Patients' fears and expectations need to be weighed during perioperative counseling. However, despite the increasing scientific interest about this topic, the evidence that can guide clinical practice is still scant and scattered.

This issue of *Thoracic Surgery Clinics* focuses on the many aspects influencing the quality of life of patients affected by surgical pulmonary diseases. Its main objective is to increase awareness about this important topic in order to promote a culture of data collection and scientific investigation ultimately leading to a better understanding of the patient perception of surgical outcome. Experts from different specialties (surgeons, chest physicians, psychologists, methodologists, physiotherapists, etc) have given their outstanding contributions to the development of this issue.

A special emphasis has been placed on lung cancer patients. The diagnosis of lung cancer determines tremendous psychosocial alterations that can even affect treatment outcome. Changes in physical and emotional aspects of quality of life need to be measured with reliable and reproducible metrics. An article has been devoted to the background and methods of the development of a quality-of-life assessment tool.

Surgery remains the mainstay of lung cancer management. Different tools have been used and published to measure the perioperative changes in quality of life. A synthesis of this evidence using a semi-quantitative and standardized approach is reported in one of the articles in this issue. The influence of minimally invasive thoracic surgery, which is increasingly used in our specialty, on residual quality of life is also discussed.

Although objective results have shown reduced morbidity and mortality in high-risk patients due to improved standards of care and technology, the impact of surgery on these high-risk patients, including those with end-stage pulmonary disease, those candidates for lung transplant, and those exposed to prolonged periods in ICU, deserves to be discussed and explored further. It is particularly in these patients that the balance between risk and benefit could be offset by the patient's opinions and preferences. For this reason specific articles have been dedicated to these subjects.

In order to have informed opinions, communication between physicians and patients is of paramount importance, particularly in a period when information is readily available in the media and Internet. An article has been entirely dedicated to the topic of communication.

The difficult job of the modern physician, who needs to integrate communication, patient information, patient expectations and opinions, and clinical decision-making, is addressed and discussed in a specific article.

The final 2 articles regard the patient's perception of the surgical outcome and the patient's safety. These 2 topics are becoming increasingly

Thorac Surg Clin 22 (2012) ix–x
http://dx.doi.org/10.1016/j.thorsurg.2012.08.002
1547-4127/12/$ – see front matter © 2012 Elsevier Inc. All rights reserved.

important in our profession, as they will influence physicians' credentialing, quality assurance, and reimbursement.

I hope the outstanding contributions collected in this issue will be useful information for both practicing physicians and investigators and contribute to increased interest and knowledge about this crucial aspect of our profession—the patient's perspective.

Alessandro Brunelli, MD
Section of Minimally Invasive Thoracic Surgery
Division of Thoracic Surgery
Ospedali Riuniti Ancona
Via Conca 1
60122 Ancona, Italy

E-mail address:
brunellialex@gmail.com

A 30-Year Perspective on Psychosocial Issues in Lung Cancer
How Lung Cancer "Came Out of the Closet"

Talia Weiss, MA[a],*, Mark Weinberger, PhD, MPH[b],
Arielle M. Schwerd, BA[c], Jimmie Holland, MD[c]

KEYWORDS

- Psychosocial issues • Lung cancer • Advocacy • Stigma

KEY POINTS

- Psychological responses to lung cancer have changed over the past 30 years as perceptions of the disease have changed.
- Previously seen as a fatal diagnosis, lung cancer is now regarded as a cancer whose treatment is increasingly effective as the science of the disease advances, particularly in regard to genetic mutations.
- Strong advocacy advances have developed nationally for patients with lung cancer.
- The increasing social support and greater knowledge of lung cancer provides a more supportive situation in which patients cope with lung cancer today, compared with 30 years ago.

"Would you believe I sit in the waiting room and wish that I had breast cancer—there is so much more support for them."
—Lung cancer patient, 1992[1]

INTRODUCTION

The psychological responses to lung cancer are strongly influenced by the perceptions of society about the disease. Cancer in general has been feared for centuries as a disease of unknown cause and largely unknown cure. Among the sites of cancer, lung has been one most feared because of the high mortality and the infrequent diagnosis at an early stage that is curable. However, added to that burden for patients with lung cancer is the onus of having "brought the disease on yourself." Although long suspected of deleterious health effects, in 1964 the Surgeon General reported the relationship between lung cancer and cigarette smoking.[2] In a country with a high percentage of smokers, this news was taken lightly because several generations of adults had grown up believing "smoking calmed the nerves" and was a sign of sophistication. Adolescents thought smoking made them look smart and grown up. Tobacco companies, representing a major industry in the United States, made smoking look glamorous in advertisement after advertisement. The immediate effect of the Surgeon General's report was a blast of cigarette company's advertisements to allay the public's fears about smoking. Much lower amounts of advertising money were available for public service announcements supporting the dangers of smoking. The public was bombarded with the 2 messages that cigarettes were safe versus those in which public health officials noted how

[a] Clinical Psychology, Health Emphasis Ferkauf Graduate School of Psychology, Yeshiva University and Memorial Sloan-Kettering Cancer Center, New York, USA; [b] IMA Clinical Research, Tarrytown, NY 10591, USA; [c] Memorial Sloan-Kettering Cancer Center, New York, USA
* Corresponding author.
E-mail address: taliarweiss@gmail.com

Thorac Surg Clin 22 (2012) 449–456
http://dx.doi.org/10.1016/j.thorsurg.2012.07.008
1547-4127/12/$ – see front matter Published by Elsevier Inc.

thoracic.theclinics.com

dangerous they were, for not only cancer of the lung but also aerodigestive and genitourinary tract, especially bladder.

The antismoking campaigns were very aggressive, and the message to people with lung cancer was "let the people presently affected with lung cancer die and just concentrate on prevention." The result was that patients with lung cancer were always asked immediately, "Did you smoke?"[3] Patients would try to avoid revealing that their site of cancer was lung because of the sense that others would blame them and that they were less deserving of sympathy than patients with cancers of other sites. They felt shame added to their own personal feelings of guilt and regret for taking up smoking. Patients with lung cancer believed that little research was being done in the treatment of lung cancer because the general opinion was that they had brought the disease on themselves. The societal views have changed as more has become known about the molecular biology of lung cancer and the increasing incidence in former and never smokers. More support services are now available for patients with lung cancer, and lung cancer has "come out of the closet" as a disease site that was once too stigmatized to even reveal.[4] Efforts to make a diagnosis at an earlier stage have increased interest in closer surveillance in people who have smoked.

Lung cancer has been described as the "unfashionable" cancer.[5] These patients have voiced their frustration and sadness regarding the stigma they face. One patient described it as the "most stigmatized, ignored, underfunded cancer of all," whereas another said, "[w]hen you discover you have it, there is a shocking stigma, there isn't a lot of support out there unfortunately."[5] Because of the strong association between smoking and lung cancer, the public perception has been that lung cancer is self-inflicted and a disease "tainted by smoking"[6] or a moral punishment.[7] One patient was saddened by the perception that patients with lung cancer who smoked are dirty and blameworthy.[8] These associations and perceptions stigmatize smokers[9–12] and people who are diagnosed with lung cancer,[5,13] and diminish sympathy for patients with lung cancer.[14,15] Graphic "quit smoking" television campaigns, however effective, in fact contribute to fear and anxiety in patients with lung cancer because of the portrayal of an unavoidable "dreadful death."[5] Stigma increases the stress associated with cancer[16–18] and contributes to psychological and social morbidity.[18,19] Patients who never smoked are quick to defend themselves, asserting they are innocent victims to distinguish themselves from smokers. This reaction has serious consequences: patients may conceal their illness,[18,20] feel "unworthy" of medical treatment,[20] delay seeking treatment,[15] and practice poor compliance.[21,22]

Cigarette smoking accounts for 85% to 90% of lung cancer; risk increases with number of packs smoked and duration of smoking.[23,24] Exposure to secondhand smoke causes approximately 3400 lung cancer deaths among nonsmokers every year.[25] Little question remains that the lung cancer epidemic relates to tobacco and the antismoking campaigns have been important. However, the backlash for patients with lung cancer was unforeseen.

A provocative advertisement campaign on behalf of the Lung Cancer Alliance was launched in June 2012 to combat the stigma. The campaign's theme, "No one Deserves to Die," addresses the "pervasive demonizing" of patients with lung cancer (**Fig. 1**). The campaign states, "Many people believe that if you have lung cancer you did something to deserve it...Lung cancer doesn't discriminate and neither should you. Help put an

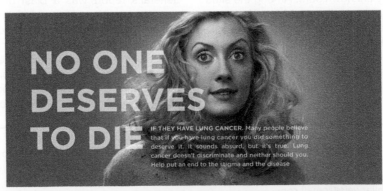

Fig. 1. Image from June 2012 "No one deserves to die" advertisement campaign on behalf of the Lung Cancer Alliance. (*Courtesy of* Lung Cancer Alliance, Washington, DC; with permission. Available at: http://noonedeservestodie.org/.).

end to the stigma and the disease."[26] Laurie Fenton Ambrose, president of the Lung Cancer Alliance, described the campaign: "This isn't a campaign about smoking. This is a campaign about the stigma and the harm it does to lung cancer patients, whether or not they've smoked. The stigma is literally the biggest obstacle in the way of achieving any progress in terms of lung cancer's survivability. Until we can get beyond that, we will never see a change."[27]

PSYCHOSOCIAL IMPACT OF LUNG CANCER

In addition to the impact of societal attitudes, patients with lung cancer also experience the usual concerns that accompany any cancer diagnosis. These factors lead to distress related to several areas: the need to cope with physical symptoms (pain, fatigue, nausea); coping with psychological concerns (eg, fears, sadness); psychiatric complications (depression, anxiety, delirium); social concerns (for family and their future); spiritual concerns (seeking comforting religious, spiritual, or philosophic beliefs); and existential concerns (seeking meaning in life while confronting death).

In the largest study of distress by cancer site (N = 4496; lung = 692), Zabora and colleagues[28] found lung cancer was the site associated with the most distress, with 43% of patients with lung cancer meeting criteria for clinically significant distress. Other studies have shown a broader range based on clinical criteria and methods: 23% to 62%.[29–33] High rates of distress occur in patients with lung cancer in palliative care (65%), likely because of psychological, social, and physical symptoms.[30] Risk factors related to higher distress are depression,[29,34] anxiety,[29,34] pain,[29,34] fatigue,[29] shortness of breath,[35] younger age,[29,34] female sex,[36] living alone,[36] and helplessness/hopelessness as a coping style.[36]

Depression is also frequent in patients with lung cancer. As cited by Shimizu and colleagues,[37] rates of clinically significant depression range from 9% to 53%.[33,34,38–48] Zabora and colleagues[28] found that patients with lung cancer had the highest mean depression score of 13 sites of cancer. Depression can result in decreased adherence to treatment; longer hospital stays[49]; difficulty making treatment decisions[50–53]; inappropriate feelings of hopelessness leading to suicidal thoughts, especially in the presence of fatigue; anorexia; and pain.[54,55]

Based on results of previous studies documented by Shimizu and colleagues,[37] risk factors for depression in patients with lung cancer are advanced cancer stage,[34,47] poor performance status,[38] younger age,[34,56] female sex,[36] living alone,[36] absence of a confidant,[36,47,57] poorer employment status,[58] lower educational status,[47] use of alcohol,[34] smoking,[59] lower body weight,[60] and physical symptoms of pain,[34] dyspnea,[61] and fatigue.[38,62] Others have found that fatigue,[35,63] weakness,[63] insomnia,[35,63] cough,[35,63] alopecia,[63] loss of appetite,[35] weight loss,[35] difficulty breathing,[35] and increased sputum[35] are related to depression.

Perceived stigma is correlated with depression and quality of life (QOL). Regardless of whether a person with lung cancer has ever smoked, lung cancer stigma has a strong positive relationship with depression and a strong inverse relationship with QOL.[64]

Rates of anxiety range from 10% to 46%.[38,63,65–67] Zabora and colleagues[28] found that patients with lung cancer had the second highest mean anxiety score. Risk factors for anxiety are fatigue,[35,63,68,69] weakness,[63] insomnia,[35,63] loss of appetite,[35] weight loss,[35] increased sputum,[35] cough,[35] and dyspnea.[35,69,70] Anxiety results in decreased adherence to treatment and longer hospital stays.[49] Anxiety is speculated to be a risk factor for suicide in patients with cancer.[71]

Carlsen and colleagues[72] noted that psychosocial well-being and QOL are significantly dependent on symptoms of lung cancer,[73] physical functioning,[73] and presence of depression.[40] Others have found that predictors of psychosocial well-being and QOL are dyspnea,[67,70] anxiety,[67] depression,[67,74] fatigue,[67,74,75] pain,[67,75] cough,[67] and decreased physical activity (in survivors).[76] A qualitative study by Berterö and colleagues[77] identified through interviews 6 themes that were major concerns impacting QOL: the experience of uncertainty, maintaining hope, concern for others providing support, thoughts of death, feelings of personal shame and sadness, and responses of family. These themes gave structure to the struggle to live as usual, maintaining independence and integrity.

LESSONS FROM THE MEMORIAL SLOAN-KETTERING CANCER CENTER LUNG CANCER SUPPORT GROUP (1992–2012)

In the early 1990s, no support groups were available in the United States for patients with lung cancer despite the fact that there was widespread support and advocacy for women with breast cancer. The quote, "Would you believe I sit in the waiting room and wish that I had *breast* cancer— there is so much more support for them" was the impetus for starting the first lung cancer support group at Memorial Sloan-Kettering Cancer Center. As a small national advocacy organization, however, it did not have the resources to reach many patients with lung cancer. At the time of the first meetings, survival from inoperable lung cancer was short. Patients felt that talking to others was a source of solace. One patient expressed it well by saying "we're all in the same leaky boat." The shared feeling of camaraderie was helpful. However, many patients could not tolerate these discussions and found the meetings too painful. They coped predominantly by not facing the reality of their situations until the level of illness required it.

Through the notes kept from these meetings, some common themes were gleaned, which are expressed by quotes from patients.[78]

The Stigma of a Lung Cancer Diagnosis

- "If one more person asks me if I smoked, I'm gonna poke them in the nose!"
- "Lung cancer is a death sentence."
- "The silence is deafening in terms of advocacy for lung cancer."
- "I don't tell people because I'm afraid if they know my diagnosis they'll treat me differently."
- "What do you say when people ask you if you smoked? You say, 'Gee, that's interesting, why do you wanna know? Do *you* smoke?'"

Insensitive Comments of Others

- "You look good, considering…"
- "If you're still around in 3 months, come see me."
- "People often have me buried while I'm still alive."
- "Families should listen and shut up. Don't tell me what to do or give me any 'shoulds.'"
- "People don't understand that I look well even though I am sick."
- "People tell you about every treatment they've heard of and it's no help."

Symptoms of Illness and Side Effects of Treatments

- "It's not the issue of dying so much as getting there and how."
- On losing one's hair: "One is never prepared for what one will look like. I thought I was prepared, but I wasn't."
- "Just the thought of so many [medications] makes me want to retch."
- "If the cancer doesn't kill you, the remedy certainly will."

- "You can be happy as long as you can breathe."
- "The idea that I'll never be able to do some things again (sailing, going to the movies) is so depressing."
- "The demons come out at night."
- "When it's hard to breathe you cannot think of anything else."

The Use of Humor

- "Humor allows you to express a lot of things you normally cannot."
- "A week before a scan of my lungs I get PSP—pre-scan psychosis—which goes away when the scan hasn't changed for the worst."
- "There is no such thing as 'minor' surgery."
- On clinical trials: "I wanna know that at least the mice did well!"
- "I eat dessert first now."
- On the positive side of chemotherapy: "Since I have been on [chemotherapy], I no longer have to shave my arms and legs, but I do miss my eyelashes!"
- "When somebody says 'my gut tells me you're gonna be ok' my reaction is: 'what does your gut know about my cancer!'"
- "Anything you find that makes you laugh is valuable."
- "I look at the [mayonnaise] jar and I wonder which will last longer."
- "First thing I did was cancel the dentist and the eye doctor."
- "At least there is one benefit of lung cancer: you can get handicapped parking."
- "Life is a highway; when you get diagnosed you merge onto the express lane."

Uncertainty

- "If you don't ask for what you want, how will your prayers be answered?"
- "Imagine the worst and hope for the best."
- "There's not a lot of time left, I don't want to waste it."
- "When you've had cancer, any time you have pain you think it's the cancer coming back. There is no such thing as a 'normal pain' or 'old age pain.'"
- "I live from one CAT scan to another."
- "Enjoy the ups. Tolerate the downs."
- "There is a cloud of uncertainty over us all."
- "Is it worth it to go through treatment only to die anyway?"
- "It's like living with a sword over your head, waiting for something to happen at any time."

- "I wonder which of us will be here for next Christmas…"
- On medical advances: "Will the breakthroughs come soon enough?"
- "Until you go through this, you cannot realize the depth of fear."
- "My doctor said to me, 'You failed the protocol' but I think the protocol failed me!"

Being a Burden on Spouse and Family

- "It's very hard to become dependent on others. Who's going to take care of my child when I'm gone?"
- "I worry about the burden on my spouse when I can't take care of myself."

Social Isolation

- "Who will take care of me if I am single and alone?"
- "Sometimes you have to be your own advocate."
- "It's hard to be sick alone."
- "One of the most important things about the support group is that I am no longer alone. It makes me feel less afraid."
- "I don't want to go out in the world because I feel as if I've just been shut out of it."

Philosophic Approaches to Coping

- "We are each a statistic of one."
- "I find I smell the roses more now that I'm ill."
- "I appreciate my family more."
- "Living with lung cancer is like living with a loaded gun pressed up against your head. How do you do it? By taking one day at a time."
- On coping with bad news: "First you fall apart and then you deal with it day by day."
- "Since my diagnosis, I have finite goals: to see my children, spend time with family, have the least amount of pain possible, and not get involved with the distractions life throws at you."
- "Don't stop enjoying life."
- "Living right doesn't protect us from bad things happening."

SUMMARY

Psychological responses to lung cancer have changed over the past 30 years as perceptions of the disease have changed. Previously seen as a fatal diagnosis, it is now regarded as a cancer whose treatment is increasingly effective as the science of the disease advances, particularly regarding genetic mutations. Strong advocacy advances have developed nationally for patients with lung cancer, and through the Lung Cancer Alliance and many foundations devoted to lung cancer research. The stigma of smoking is diminishing as more is learned about genetic factors and as more nonsmokers are diagnosed. Support groups are available in most cities, online (www.cancersupportcommunity.org, www.lungevity.org, www.acor.org), and through telephone resources (Lung Cancer Alliance Phone Buddy Program; 800-298-2436). A national toll-free helpline (866-276-7443) exists to help patients find a counselor in their own community. The increasing social support and greater knowledge of lung cancer provide a more supportive environment in which patients cope with lung cancer today compared with 30 years ago.

ACKNOWLEDGMENTS

The authors wish to express gratitude for the contributions of Elizabeth Peabody, LMSW, who co-led the group for more than 20 years and diligently kept notes at our twice-monthly Lung Cancer Support Group. We would also like to thank Elizabeth Blackler, LMSW, who has served as the co-leader of the group for the past 3 years.

REFERENCES

1. Holland J, Lewis S. The human side of cancer. New York: Harper Collins; 1999.
2. Advisory Committee to the Surgeon General of the Public Health Service. The reports of the surgeon general: smoking and health. 1964. Available at: http://profiles.nlm.nih.gov/NN/B/B/M/Q/. Accessed July 1, 2012.
3. Holland JC, Kelly BJ, Weinberger MI. Why psychosocial care is difficult to integrate into routine cancer care: stigma is the elephant in the room. J Natl Compr Canc Netw 2010;8:362–6.
4. Patterson JT. The dread disease: cancer and modern American culture. Cambridge (MA): Harvard University Press; 1989.
5. Chapple A, Ziebland S, McPherson A. Stigma, shame, and blame experienced by patients with lung cancer: qualitative study. BMJ 2004;328(7454):1470.
6. American Cancer Society. Many Lung Cancer Patients Feel Stigmatized Even Non-Smokers Feel Blame, Guilt [report on the Internet]. Altanta (GA); 2004. Available at: http://archive.tobacco.org/news/167876.html.
7. Unger M. A pause, progress, and reassessment in lung cancer screening. N Engl J Med 2006;355:1822–4.

8. Conlon A, Gilbert D, Jones B, et al. Stacked stigma: oncology social workers' perceptions of the lung cancer experience. J Psychosoc Oncol 2010;28: 98–115.

9. Kim SH, Shanahan J. Stigmatizing smokers: public sentiment toward cigarette smoking and its relationship to smoking behaviors. J Health Commun 2003; 8:343–67.

10. Bell K, Salmon A, Bowers M, et al. Smoking, stigma and tobacco 'denormalization': further reflections on the use of stigma as a public health tool. A commentary on social science & medicine's stigma, prejudice, discrimination and health special issue. Soc Sci Med 2010;67:795–9.

11. Burris S. Stigma, ethics and policy: a commentary on Bayer's "stigma and the ethics of public health: not can we but should we". Soc Sci Med 2008;67: 473–5.

12. Rozin P, Singh L. The moralization of cigarette smoking in the United States. J Consum Psychol 1999;8:321–37.

13. Lebel S, Devins GM. Stigma in cancer patients whose behaviour may have contributed to their disease. Future Oncol 2008;4:717–33.

14. Wakefield M, McLeod K, Smith K. Individual versus corporate responsibility for smoking-related illness: Australian press coverage of the Rolah McCabe trial. Health Promot Int 2003;18:297–305.

15. MacKenzie R, Chapman S, Holding S. Framing responsibility: coverage of lung cancer among smokers and non-smokers in Australian television news. Aust N Z J Public Health 2011;35(1):66–70.

16. Carmack C, Badr H, Lee J, et al. Lung cancer patients and their spouses: psychological and relation- ship functioning within one month of treatment initiation. Ann Behav Med 2008;36: 129–40.

17. Marlow L, Waller L, Wardle J. Variation in blame attributions across different cancer types. Cancer Epidemiol Biomarkers Prev 2010;19:1799–805.

18. Berterö C. Living with social anguish: shame and guilt in lung cancer patients. OASJ 2008;1:26–30.

19. Lebel S, Castonguay M, Mackness G, et al. The psychosocial impact of stigma in people with head and neck or lung cancer. Psychooncology 2011. http://dx.doi.org/10.1002/pon.2063.

20. Corner J, Hopkinson J, Roffe L. Experience of health changes and reasons for delay in seeking care: a UK study of the months prior to the diagnosis of lung cancer. Soc Sci Med 2006;62:1381–91.

21. Sher I, McGinn L, Sirey JA, et al. Effects of caregivers' perceived stigma and causal beliefs on patients' adherence to antidepressant treatment. Psychiatr Serv 2005;56:564–9.

22. LoConte NK, Else-Quest NM, Eickhoff J, et al. Assessment of guilt and shame in patients with non–small-cell lung cancer compared with patients with breast and prostate cancer. Clin Lung Cancer 2008; 9:171–8.

23. Carmona R. The Health Consequences of Smoking. A Report of the U.S. Surgeon General. Atlanta (Ga): U.S. Department of Health and Human Services; 2004.

24. Cooley ME, Lynch J, Fox K, et al. Lung cancer. In: Holland JC, Breitbart WS, Jacobsen PB, et al, editors. Psycho-Oncology. 2nd edition. New York: Oxford University Press; 2010. p. 152–9.

25. Lloyd AC, Denton JE. Identification of environmental tobacco smoke as a toxic air contaminant. Executive Summary. Sacramento (Ca): California Environmental Protection Agency; 2005.

26. Lung Cancer Alliance. Available at: http:// noonedeservestodie.org/. Accessed July 1, 2012.

27. Elliot S. Cancer campaign tries using shock to change attitudes. New York Times 2012. Available at: http://www.nytimes.com/2012/07/09/business/media/cancer-campaign-tries-using-shock-to-change-attitudes-campaign-spotlight.html?_r=2&adxnnl=1&pagewanted=all&adxnnlx=1346155746-5GgI61-DEm3JSHDIDTNFHsg. Accessed August 28, 2012.

28. Zabora J, BrintzenhofeSzoc K, Curbow B, et al. The prevalence of psychological distress by cancer site. Psychooncology 2001;10:19–28.

29. Graves KD, Arnold SM, Love CL, et al. Distress screening in a multidisciplinary lung cancer clinic: prevalence and predictors of clinically significant distress. Lung Cancer 2007;55:215–24.

30. Wei Gao W, Bennett MI, Stark DS, et al. Psychological distress in cancer from survivorship to end of life care: prevalence, associated factors and clinical implications. Eur J Cancer 2010;46:2036–44.

31. Carlson LE, Groff SL, Maciejewski O, et al. Screening for distress in lung and breast cancer outpatients: a randomized controlled trial. J Clin Oncol 2010;28:4884–91.

32. Steinberg T, Roseman M, Kasymjanova G, et al. Prevalence of emotional distress in newly diagnosed lung cancer patients. Support Care Cancer 2009;17: 1493–7.

33. Sanders SL, Bantum EO, Owen JE, et al. Supportive care needs in patients with lung cancer. Psychooncology 2010;19:480–9.

34. Akechi T, Okamura H, Nishiwaki Y, et al. Psychiatric disorders and associated and predictive factors in patients with unresectable nonsmall cell lung carcinoma: a longitudinal study. Cancer 2001;92:2609–22.

35. Kuo TT, Ma FC. Symptom distresses and coping strategies in patients with non-small cell lung cancer. Cancer Nurs 2002;25:309–17.

36. Akechi T, Kugaya A, Okamura H, et al. Predictive factors for psychological distress in ambulatory lung cancer patients. Support Care Cancer 1998;6: 281–6.

37. Shimizu K, Nakaya N, Saito-Nakaya K, et al. Clinical biopsychosocial risk factors for depression in lung cancer patients: a comprehensive analysis using data from the Lung Cancer Database Project. Ann Oncol 2012;23(8):1973–9.

38. Hopwood P, Stephens RJ. Depression in patients with lung cancer: prevalence and risk factors derived from quality-of-life data. J Clin Oncol 2000; 18:893–903.

39. Hyodo I, Eguchi K, Takigawa N, et al. Psychological impact of informed consent in hospitalized cancer patients. A sequential study of anxiety and depression using the hospital anxiety and depression scale. Support Care Cancer 1998;7:396–9.

40. Montazeri A, Milroy R, Hole D, et al. Anxiety and depression in patients with lung cancer before and after diagnosis: findings from a population in Glasgow, Scotland. J Epidemiol Community Health 1998;52:203–4.

41. Turner NJ, Muers MF, Haward RA, et al. Psychological distress and concerns of elderly patients treated with palliative radiotherapy for lung cancer. Psychooncology 2007;16:707–13.

42. Buccheri G. Depressive reactions to lung cancer are common and often followed by a poor outcome. Eur Respir J 1998;11:173–8.

43. Walker CC, Salinas KA, Harris PS, et al. A proteomic (SELDI-TOF-MS) approach to estrogen agonist screening. Toxicol Sci 2007;95:74–81.

44. Kurtz ME, Kurtz JC, Stommel M, et al. Predictors of depressive symptomatology of geriatric patients with lung cancer—a longitudinal analysis. Psychoon-cology 2002;11:12–22.

45. Berard RM, Boermeester F, Viljoen G. Depressive disorders in an out-patient oncology setting: prevalence, assessment, and management. Psychooncology 1998;7:112–20.

46. Tagay S, Herpertz S, Langkafel M, et al. Health-related quality of life, depression and anxiety in thyroid cancer patients. Qual Life Res 2006;15:695–703.

47. Uchitomi Y, Mikami I, Nagai K, et al. Depression and psychological distress in patients during the year after curative resection of non-small-cell lung cancer. J Clin Oncol 2003;21:69–77.

48. Suzuki S, Akechi T, Kobayashi M, et al. Daily omega-3 fatty acid intake and depression in Japanese patients with newly diagnosed lung cancer. Br J Cancer 2004;90:787–93.

49. Miller K, Massie MJ. Depressive disorders. In: Holland J, Breitbart W, Jacobsen PB, et al, editors. Psycho-Oncology. 2nd edition. New York: Oxford University Press; 2010. p. 311–8.

50. Reynolds CF, Dew MA, Pollock BG, et al. Maintenance treatment of major depression in old age. N Engl J Med 2006;354:1130–8.

51. Katon W, Lin E, Kroenke K. The association of depression and anxiety with medical symptom burden in patients with chronic medical illness. Gen Hosp Psychiatry 2007;29(2):147–55.

52. Katon W, Sullivan M. Depression and chronic medical illness. J Clin Psychiatry 1990;51:3–34.

53. Katon WJ, Schoenbaum M, Fan MY, et al. Cost-effectiveness of improving primary care treatment of late-life depression. Arch Gen Psychiatry 2005; 62(12):1313–20.

54. Henriksson MM, Isometsa ET, Hietanen PS, et al. Mental disorders in cancer suicides. J Affect Disord 1995;36:11–20.

55. Akechi T, Okamura H, Nishiwaki Y, et al. Predictive factors for suicidal ideation in patients with unresect-able lung carcinoma. Cancer 2002;92:2609–22.

56. Lo C, Zimmermann C, Rydall A, et al. Longitudinal study of depressive symptoms in patients with metastatic gastrointestinal and lung cancer. J Clin Oncol 2010;28:3084–9.

57. Uchitomi Y, Mikami I, Kugaya A, et al. Physician support and patient psychologic responses after surgery for nonsmall cell lung carcinoma: a prospective observational study. Cancer 2001;92:1926–35.

58. Agarwal M, Hamilton JB, Moore CE, et al. Predictors of depression among older African American cancer patients. Cancer Nurs 2010;33:156–63.

59. Schnoll RA, Malstrom M, James C, et al. Correlates of tobacco use among smokers and recent quitters diagnosed with cancer. Patient Educ Couns 2002; 46:137–45.

60. Lasheen W, Walsh D. The cancer anorexia-cachexia syndrome: myth or reality? Support Care Cancer 2010;18:265–72.

61. Tanaka K, Akechi T, Okuyama T, et al. Factors correlated with dyspnea in advanced lung cancer patients: organic causes and what else? J Pain Symptom Manage 2002;23:490–500.

62. Okuyama T, Tanaka K, Akechi T, et al. Fatigue in ambulatory patients with advanced lung cancer: prevalence, correlated factors, and screening. J Pain Symptom Manage 2001;22:554–64.

63. Liao YC, Liao WY, Shun SC, et al. Symptoms, psychological distress, and supportive care needs in lung cancer patients. Support Care Cancer 2011;19:1743–51.

64. Cataldo JK, Jahan TM, Pongquan VL. Lung cancer stigma, depression, and quality of life among ever and never smokers. Eur J Oncol Nurs 2012;16:264–9.

65. Rolke HB, Bakke PS, Gallefoss F. Health related quality of life, mood disorders and coping abilities in an unselected sample of patients with primary lung cancer. Respir Med 2008;102:1460–7.

66. Wiljer D, Walton T, Gilbert J, et al. Understanding the needs of lung cancer patients during the pre-diagnosis phase. J Canc Educ 2012;27:494–500.

67. Henoch I, Bergman B, Gustafsson M, et al. The impact of symptoms, coping capacity, and social support on quality of life experience over time in

patients with lung cancer. J Pain Symptom Manage 2007;34:370–9.

68. Brown DJ, McMillan DC, Milroy R. The correlation between fatigue, physical function, the systemic inflammatory response, and psychological distress in patients with advanced lung cancer. Cancer 2005;103(2):377–82.

69. Chan CH, Richardson A, Janet Richardson J. Managing symptoms in patients with advanced lung cancer during radiotherapy: results of a psychoeducational randomized controlled trial. J Pain Symptom Manage 2011;41:347–57.

70. Smith EL, Hann DM, Ahles TA, et al. Dyspnea, anxiety, body consciousness, and quality of life in patients with lung cancer. J Pain Symptom Manage 2001;21:323–9.

71. Levin T, Alici Y. Anxiety disorders. In: Holland JC, editor. Psycho-oncology. 2nd edition. New York: Oxford University Press; 2010. p. 324–31.

72. Carlsen K, Jensen AB, Jacobsen E, et al. Psychosocial aspects of lung cancer. Lung Cancer 2005;47: 293–300.

73. Kaasa S, Mastekaasa A. Psychosocial well-being of patients with inoperable non-small cell lung cancer: the importance of treatment- and disease-related factors. Acta Oncol 1998;27:829–35.

74. Fox SW, Lyon DE. Symptom clusters and quality of life in survivors of lung cancer. Oncol Nurs Forum 2006;33:931–6.

75. Braun DP, Gupta D, Staren ED. Quality of life assessment as a predictor of survival in non-small cell lung cancer. BMC Cancer 2011;11:353.

76. Nes LS, Liu H, Patten CA, et al. Physical activity level and quality of life in long term lung cancer survivors. Lung Cancer 2012;77(3):611–6.

77. Bertero C, Vanhanen M, Appelin G. Receiving a diagnosis of inoperable lung cancer: patients' perspectives of how it affects their life situation and quality of life. Acta Oncol 2008;47:862–9.

78. Holland J, Peabody E, Blackler E. Changing concerns among patients with advanced lung cancer: themes which stay the same and those that change. Psychooncology 2010;19(suppl 1): S1–102.

Quality of Life in Pulmonary Surgery
Choosing, Using, and Developing Assessment Tools

D. Fitzsimmons, PhD[a], S. Wheelwright, MA[b], C.D. Johnson, FRCS[b,*]

KEYWORDS

- Health-related quality of life • Lung • Pulmonary • Surgery • Assessment • Review

KEY POINTS

- Careful attention must be paid when choosing, using, and developing health-related quality of life (HRQOL) assessment tools in pulmonary surgery populations.
- Although choice is still limited, there is increasing attention paid to the specific HRQOL considerations for different pulmonary surgical populations.
- A review of recent studies in patients with lung cancer undergoing surgical intervention has identified common limitations in using HRQOL assessment tools.
- New developments with the field are providing better ways to ensure HRQOL assessment places the patient perspective at the center of surgical decision making.

INTRODUCTION

Quality of life (QOL) has received increasing attention in evaluating surgical interventions for pulmonary disease, in line with a general increasing need and demand to consider the patient perspective.

QOL is a general term that spans a range of topics.[1] The challenge in making a broad reference to QOL is that it is an abstract concept that is subjective and individual and depends on a person's circumstances. The focus of clinical research has been on assessing health-related quality of life (HRQOL). Although not without criticism,[2] it has allowed focus on assessing areas of QOL that can be reasonably influenced by disease and its treatments.[3]

There has been mounting recognition that treatment efficacy needs to be measured in a variety of ways, with HRQOL now widely regarded as an important outcome. Understanding the outcome of treatment from the viewpoint of the patient is central to evaluating the quality of health care[4] and capturing the essence of patient-centered care,[5] with such information having the potential to make a vital contribution to clinical decision making for individual patients[6] right through to national guidance on what represents the most clinically effective and cost-effective treatment.[7–9]

For patients with pulmonary disease, surgical interventions may confer a range of benefits including improved survival, symptom improvement, and improvements in HRQOL. However, surgery may also result in postoperative mortality, morbidity, and impairment in HRQOL. The short- and long-term effects of surgery on a patient's HRQOL must be considered.[10] As surgical techniques advance and patients become more involved in treatment decisions, robust information is required from the patient perspective.[5]

[a] Swansea Centre for Health Economics, College of Human and Health Sciences, Swansea University, Singleton Park, Swansea, SA2 8PP, United Kingdom; [b] University Surgical Unit, University of Southampton School of Medicine, Southampton University Hospital, Tremona Road, Southampton, S016 6YD, United Kingdom
* Corresponding author. University Surgical Unit, Southampton University Hospital, Tremona Road, Southampton SO16 6YD, UK.
E-mail address: c.d.johnson@soton.ac.uk

Thorac Surg Clin 22 (2012) 457–470
http://dx.doi.org/10.1016/j.thorsurg.2012.07.007
1547-4127/12/$ – see front matter © 2012 Elsevier Inc. All rights reserved.

However, HRQOL is not a "one-size-fits-all" solution to incorporating the patient perspective in pulmonary surgery. Different approaches and methods to HRQOL assessment are required in different contexts, and each approach requires a well-designed and validated assessment tool to provide clinically useful information.[6,11]

Everyone involved in the design, conduct, and interpretation of surgical trials and studies must become familiar with the methods and techniques used in HRQOL assessment.[5] This is essential because HRQOL assessment must stand up to the same scientific scrutiny as other outcome measures; that is, it should provide a relevant, valid, measurable endpoint that provides clinically meaningful information on the risks or benefits of pulmonary surgery. In this review, the authors aim to provide a comprehensive overview of the key issues to consider if an investigator wishes to incorporate HRQOL assessment into trials and studies of pulmonary surgery, drawing on recent studies of lung cancer surgery as an example.

Therapeutic Options

Selecting HRQOL as an outcome of concern for trials and studies in pulmonary surgery

There are increasing numbers of studies reporting HRQOL in patients with pulmonary disease. However, the "popularity" of HRQOL should not be used as the only justification for its inclusion.

The questions to ask are, Is HRQOL is an appropriate endpoint? Should it be a primary or secondary endpoint? There will be several factors influencing the answers to these 2 questions, including what are the expected benefits of the treatment and intervention and, of importance, what outcomes are considered to be most important and relevant from the patient perspective. Survival will continue to be the primary endpoint for pulmonary surgery when treatment is curative or potentially curative or when long-term survival is expected. However, HRQOL may complement this by considering the quality of the patient's survival.[12] The challenges faced during the postoperative period can result in short- and long-term problems,[10] and any survival benefit needs to be considered in the context of impact on patient function and HRQOL.[13–15] In pulmonary surgery with palliative intent, HRQOL may be the main endpoint of concern.[16]

Clinical Outcomes

Choosing an HRQOL assessment approach

Once the decision is made to include an HRQOL assessment, a careful decision must be made on whether to use an already available assessment tool, to adapt an existing tool, or to develop a new assessment tool. Insufficient consideration of whether an assessment tool actually measures those HRQOL issues that the study team (and, more important, the patient) considers significant and relevant can result in the selection of an assessment tool that provides inadequate or inaccurate information. As demonstrated in systematic reviews of other surgical populations, the consequence of poor or limited HRQOL assessment can result in limited interpretations being drawn from studies reporting HRQOL.[14,16,17]

Types of HRQOL assessments

A patient-reported outcome measurement (PROM) is the assessment of any aspect of a patient's health status that is reported by the patient themselves, without interpretation from a clinician about what they think in relation to a health condition and its treatment.[18,19] With this broad term, PROMs focus on symptoms and treatment side effects, functional limitations, and satisfaction with care, as well as more complex concepts such as HRQOL.[19] HRQOL assessment tools can be divided into 2 main types: preference-based and profile (non–preference)-based assessment.

Preference-based HRQOL assessments Preference-based HRQOL assessments are used in economic evaluation (cost-utility analysis). The HRQOL assessment must generate a weight or utility value giving a score between 1 (representing full health) and 0 (representing death).[6,20] This indicates a preference for different health states that are more desirable. Utilities can be derived from direct methods such as time tradeoff or standard gamble directs or indirect methods, with an HRQOL assessment tool, that can be used to generate a utility score based on values, usually obtained from general population samples.[20,21] Common examples of generic HRQOL tools are the EQ-5D[22] and (SF)6D.[23] Condition-specific measures are sometimes available, such as the Asthma Quality of Life Questionnaire[24] (for which scores need to be mapped across to a generic measure) or a measure developed from the European Organisation for Research and Treatment for Cancer Quality of Life Questionnaire (EORTC QLQ-C30) for cancer populations.[25] Although there is no doubt that preference-based HRQOL assessment is extremely important, the authors focus on profile-based HRQOL assessment, which is more useful for assessing individual patient outcomes.

Profile-based HRQOL assessments Profile-based HRQOL assessments are used to capture HRQOL information, usually across several domains. Although every assessment tool will differ in the domains that are included, several common domains are often covered (**Table 1**), depending on the purpose of the tool.

Typically, a patient is asked to rate his or her response (eg, extent to which the patient has experienced a specific problem) based on a Likert scale. The time frame on which the patient is asked to rate the QOL can vary (eg, during the past week or month). A profile of scores is generated for either single items or scales (a group of conceptually similar [equivalent] items that assess 1 domain) or, in some cases, scores can be additionally combined into a summary score. An example is the SF-36,[26] which can provide a score across 8 different dimensions (eg, social functioning, physical functioning, and vitality) but can also provide a summary across broad domains of physical and mental health components.

HRQOL assessment is based on psychometrics (measurement theory), with properties such as validity and reliability essential ingredients[27] in determining sufficient scientific robustness of the HRQOL assessment tool. In addition, the practical issues of using HRQOL assessments must be considered. There is little point in producing the most psychometrically robust instrument that cannot be used practically because it is too long or too difficult for a patient to complete. Several reviews have been published[28–30] that consider the key criteria in selecting an HRQOL assessment tool. A summary of the key issues in selecting an HRQOL assessment tool is presented in **Table 2**.

There are 3 main types of profile HRQOL measures: generic, dimension specific, and disease specific. Generic measures, such as the SF-36,[26] cover broad aspects of HRQOL and can be used across different diseases and treatment populations; thus allowing a common comparison of HRQOL. The main disadvantage is they often do not include specific issues of concern so they may be insensitive to the most important changes in HRQOL in a particular disease. Although less often used in clinical trials, dimension-specific measures such as the Hospital Anxiety and Depression Score (HADS)[31] focus on 1 domain of symptoms or HRQOL. They are often used with generic measures. Disease-specific measures are developed for particular patient populations and so have the advantage of being more sensitive to the needs and concerns of a specific patient population. Consequently, they lack the ability to compare across different patient populations. Examples of disease-specific HRQOL measures include the St George's Respiratory Questionnaire[32] and Chronic Respiratory Questionnaire,[33] which have been used across pulmonary patient populations, and the Functional Assessment of Cancer Therapy-Lung (FACT-L)[34] and EORTC Quality of Life Questionnaire (QLQ)-C30 and QLQ-LC13.[35]

Selecting an HRQOL assessment tool

The next question should be, Is there an HRQOL assessment tool already available for use? The authors advise that, wherever possible, a validated assessment tool that is already available should be used, on conceptual, methodologic, and practical grounds, as outlined in a recent editorial by Juniper.[36] Before the development of a new assessment tool, there needs to be a strong justification made that there is no tool currently available that can be used (or adapted). This requires thorough, systematic interrogation of the HRQOL literature in that particular patient population.

A first glance of the literature reveals a bewildering array of HRQOL assessment tools to choose from, across the spectrum of pulmonary patient populations. For example, the St George's Respiratory Questionnaire[34] has been used in patients with lung volume reduction surgery for advanced emphysema,[37] the EORTC QLQ-C30 and QLQ-LC13[35] have been used to compare different surgical techniques for pneumothorax,[38] and the SF-36[26] has been used in lung transplant patients.[39] Such instruments should be tested and challenged against the key considerations outlined in **Table 2**.

Although there is a body of literature that contains reviews of different HRQOL assessment tools across a variety of pulmonary populations (eg, pulmonary arterial hypertension,[40] interstitial lung disease,[41] pulmonary fibrosis,[42] chronic obstructive pulmonary disease[43]), less attention

Table 1
Examples of HRQOL domains covered in assessment tools

Domain	Selected Examples
Disease symptoms and treatment side effects	Pain, fatigue, dyspnea, constipation, nausea and vomiting
Physical	Mobility, self-care, activities of daily living
Psychological	Depression, anxiety, body image, coping
Cognitive	Memory loss, concentration, confusion
Social	Hobbies and interests, personal relationships, social isolation
Occupational	Work activities, financial status
Global assessments	Health, quality of life

Table 2
Overview of key issues to consider when selecting an HRQOL assessment tool

Purpose/aim	Is the rationale for assessing HRQOL clear? Is HRQOL a primary or secondary endpoint? Does the definition of HRQOL to be used in the trial fit with the conceptual basis of the selected HRQOL assessment tool?
Study population	Can HRQOL be collected by a patient-self reported measure? Are there specific demographic issues to be considered (eg, age, education level, language, cultural issues)? Does the HRQOL consider patient burden (eg, time taken to complete)? Have patient representatives been included in the choice of HRQOL assessment (eg, to ensure appropriateness, identify potential difficulties)?
Measurement properties	Have the following properties been documented? Internal consistency Test-retest reliability Interrater or intrarater reliability (if applicable) Content validity Construct validity Criterion validity (if applicable) Cross-cultural validity (if applicable) Responsiveness of the HRQOL issue to expected changes
Study design issues	Does the HRQOL assessment tool require permission for its use? Are there sufficient resources available to undertake HRQOL assessment (eg, cost of the assessment tool, staff resources, consumables)? Are there training issues for staff in administrating the HRQOL assessment tool? What is the mode of HRQOL assessment (eg, self-completion, interview administration)? When should the HRQOL assessments be done (eg, baseline, end of trial)? Has a sample size calculation been undertaken on the HRQOL assessment including adjustment for attrition?
Scoring	Does the HRQOL assessment provide an overall summary, scales, and/or single items? Can scores be interpreted (eg, minimally important difference/clinical significant difference)? Is a scoring system available; is it easy to administer? Are reference values available?
Data analysis	Has HRQOL analysis followed in accordance with the trial/study protocol? Have methods for handling missing data been considered?

has been given to specific issues in specific surgical populations. A systematic review of HRQOL measures in lung cancer could not identify any surgical populations,[44] yet several important HRQOL questions arise in patients who undergo lung surgery for cancer.[45] However, recent reviews suggest that the evidence base is developing.[46,47]

Drawing on recent studies published in lung cancer surgical populations, the authors illustrate the issues and challenges to HRQOL assessment in pulmonary surgical populations.

Complications and Concerns

HRQOL assessment in lung cancer resection
Review methods The authors undertook a structured review of the literature on PubMed for studies published between January 1, 2004, and March 31, 2012, using MeSH terms to capture *HRQOL, lung neoplasm,* and *surgery and measurement* based on a search strategy used previously.[47] Full articles were retrieved when (1) HRQOL was the main aim of the report; (2) information about the HRQOL assessment tool and methods used was presented; and (3) findings reported HRQOL scores in detail, which were specific to surgical populations only. Although not a full systematic review, this provides a comprehensive overview of recent articles reporting HRQOL in lung cancer surgery.

Results The authors identified 18 articles reporting the use of HRQOL measures[48–65] and 1 article[66] reporting psychometric validation of established

HRQOL measures. These studies demonstrated variation in study population, but common features across studies were evident (eg, in comparing surgical techniques). Only 1 study[51] reported HRQOL as a secondary outcome from a randomized controlled trial. This lack of surgical trials reporting HRQOL data is a persistent issue.[6,17]

The current findings are similar to those of other reviews of HRQOL outcomes after resection for lung cancer.[4,10,67] Studies showed different results in preoperative HRQOL scores, the duration of postoperative decline in HRQOL or whether it can return to preoperative levels; and the impact of potential covariates on HRQOL changes such as age. Although beyond the scope of the present review to debate at length, one of the key questions is whether such studies can be subjected to meta-analysis to robustly synthesize these results. An attempt to synthesize such data for lung volume reduction surgery[68] showed that HRQOL assessment was too heterogeneous for meta-analysis. The authors concentrate on reporting the quality of HRQOL assessment undertaken (**Table 3**).

The current review identified that there seems to be some emerging consistency in the assessment tools being used, with the SF-36[55–63] and EORTC QLQ-C30 and QLQ-LC13[48] emerging as the generic and disease-specific tools most often used, with 2 studies that use other measures.[56,65] The use of the SF-36 and EORTC QLQ-C30 and QLQ-LC13 was recommended in a previous systematic review[69] of PROMs in lung cancer studies. That review also recommended the FACT-L,[34] although the authors found no studies using this measure. Only 1 study was found that had specifically compared HRQOL instruments.[66] The SF-36 and EORTC QLQ-C30 and QLQ-LC13 were compared with assessment of whether these tools could detect perioperative changes in HRQOL. Low correlations were found between conceptually similar scales, suggesting that the SF-36 and EORTC QLQ assessment are measuring different aspects of HRQOL, with only emotional functioning scales having a moderate-strong correlation (>.5). Both assessments showed poor correlations with objective perioperative changes such as functional expiratory volume in one second. The authors concluded that although the 2 instruments performed similarly, the EORTC assessment provides a more detailed examination of specific thoracic symptoms. However, the results should be interpreted with caution because of the small sample, lack of follow-up evaluation, and lack of attention to other important psychometric and practical considerations.

Discussion of review findings A move to standardized HRQOL assessment will assist in making comparisons between studies, and this is now being advocated as important in raising the quality of surgical trials[70] with the development of a specific Consolidate Standards Of Reporting Trials (CONSORT) statement extension for reporting HRQOL in trials in progress.[71] However, a common limitation was the lack of an operational definition of HRQOL to support the choice of assessment tool or the consideration of potential covariates (eg, comorbidity or preoperative pulmonary function) that may influence HRQOL. Another limitation is the timing of assessments, with few studies justifying the time points chosen (eg, when postoperative effects are likely to be most problematic or when recovery is expected from complications and side effects that may affect HRQOL). Frequently, studies did not have sufficient follow-up. When longer follow-up had been undertaken, there were varying periods between assessments.

One of the issues in assessing HRQOL changes is the influence of response shift over time. A response shift is when changes occur in a patient's internal valuation placed on individual HRQOL domains as a result of change in circumstances or different perception.[72] An example is an individual who has developed an effective coping strategy to deal with a symptom such as dyspnea. This may be useful in understanding some of the apparent inconsistencies between clinical measures, such as pulmonary function and HRQOL changes. Further examination of the impact of long-term survivorship on HRQOL will be an important area for the future.[73,74]

Other limitations include small sample size, particularly when there is an attempt to measure HRQOL differences between groups, examine HRQOL changes over time, or undertake analysis to adjust for the effects of other potential covariates on HRQOL scores. The effect sizes of HRQOL scores are often small to moderate, and there has been increasing attention given to determine what should be counted as a minimally important difference.[75]

One of the persistent issues for most studies was the lack of attention paid to missing data. Patients may be lost to follow-up as a result of advancing disease or deterioration in HRQOL. Failure to include these patients in the analyses will result in biased estimates of HRQOL benefits.[76] Similar to other reviews,[14,16,17,45–47,67] the current review confirms the varying quality in the analysis and interpretation of HRQOL data.

The specific HRQOL concerns for the older surgical patient

Several studies focused on HRQOL in specific relation to the older surgical patient. This is

Table 3
Overview of studies reporting HRQOL assessment in lung cancer surgical patients

Author, Year	Study Aim/Design	Summary of Common Issues Identified
Disease-specific HRQOL assessment (EORTC QLQ-C30 and LC13)		
Balducyck et al,[48] 2007	Prospective 1-y study of 100 patients receiving lobectomy, pneumonectomy, or wedge resection	Small sample size[49,50,56,65]
		Small sample size for subgroup analysis[48,52–55,63]
Balducyck et al,[49] 2008	Prospective 1-y study of 30 patients receiving lobectomy or pneumonectomy	Lack of information on how missing data were analyzed /impact on estimation of HRQOL effects[48,49,51–55,58,59,61,62,65,100]
Balducyck et al,[50] 2009	Prospective 1-y study of 60 septuagenarians receiving lobectomy or pneumonectomy	Lack of adjustment for covariates[48–50,54,56,60,63,64]
Kenny et al,[51] 2008	Prospective 2-y evaluation of HRQOL in 130 operable patients participating in a randomized trial of positive emission tomography in preoperative assessment	Heterogeneity in lung cancer types included[57]
		Lack of oldest-old include in age comparisons[53,59]
Schulte et al,[52] 2009	Prospective 2-y study of 159 patients receiving bilobectomy/lobectomy or pneumonectomy	Short time frame of follow-up[55,58,60,62–64]
		Lack of interim postoperative assessment[57,58]
Schulte et al,[53] 2010	Prospective 2-y study of 131 patients receiving lobectomy or bilobectomy with comparison of <70 y vs >70 y with age-matched reference population	Retrospective design may have introduced recall/selection bias[56]
		Limited use of HRQOL measure in previous lung cancer surgical studies[56,65]
Win et al,[54] 2005	Prospective 6-mo study of 110 patients receiving lobectomy or pneumonectomy	Rationale of timing of HRQOL unclear[52,58,61,63–65]
Generic HRQOL assessment (SF-36)		
Brunelli et al,[55] 2007	Prospective 3-mo follow-up of 156 patients receiving lobectomy or pneumonectomy	
Handy et al,[56] 2010	Retrospective analysis of HRQOL at baseline and 6-mo follow-up in 241 patients receiving open lobectomy or	

video-assisted thoracic surgery (Ferran and Power QLI also included)

Heuker et al,[57] 2011 — Retrospective follow-up of 23 survivors >36 mo following extensive surgical resection

Moller and Sartiby,[58] 2010 — Prospective 6-mo study of 249 patients with age comparison of <70 y vs >70 y compared with age- and sex-matched reference population.

Moller and Sartiby,[59] 2012 — Long-term follow-up of Moller et al study[58] in 166 patients

Pompili et al,[60] 2011 — Prospective 3-mo study of 172 patients after lobectomy or pneumonectomy

Sarna et al,[61] 2010 — Prospective 6-mo follow-up of 119 disease-free women who received a lobectomy >6 mo to 6 y after diagnosis

Salati et al,[62] 2009 — Prospective 3-mo study in 279 patients with age-related comparison following major lung resection

Sartipy,[63] 2009 — Prospective 6-mo study in 127 patients undergoing lobectomy or pneumonectomy

Sartipy,[64] 2010 — Prospective study of 249 patients undergoing lobectomy or pneumonectomy with sex comparison and reference to age- and sex-matched reference population

Other HRQOL assessment tool

Illonen et al,[65] 2010 — Prospective 4-y study in 53 patients undergoing lobectomy or bilobectomy compared with age-standardized population (using the E15D HRQOL measure: profile and preference based)

important because it is increasingly accepted that chronologic age should not be the deciding factor when assessing a patient's fitness for surgery, with evidence emerging that older patients can tolerate surgery if accurate assessments of risk are made.[77,78] However, evidence is mounting that older people represent a distinct group in terms of their HRQOL and that there are inconsistencies in studies as identified in the authors' previous systematic review.[47] The importance of age-related differences warrants further attention.

The authors coordinated an international program to specifically address the development of an HRQOL assessment system for older patients,[79] resulting in the development of the EORTC QLQ-ELD15, which was designed for use with the EORTC QLQ-C3O in patients with cancer who were older than 70 years. The EORTC QLQ-ELD15 could be a useful measure in future evaluations of surgery in populations of older patients with lung cancer, with scope for further assessment of its use in other older populations undergoing thoracic surgery.

Developing an HRQOL assessment tool

The time and resources required to develop an HRQOL assessment tool should not be underestimated. In most cases, this process takes several years, particularly if being developed for use in several countries. There is now a demand for robust and standardized processes to be followed in PROM assessment, as exemplified by the US Food and Drug Administration and European Medical Regulatory authorities.[9,80–82]

The establishment of a research team across the different clinical and academic disciplines to support HRQOL development and the incorporation of users in the design of HRQOL assessment from the start are strongly recommended. The authors outline the key phases in development, based on the methods described in the EORTC Quality of life Group guidelines for QOL questionnaire development.[83]

Phase 1: generation of HRQOL issues

The purpose of phase 1 is to establish and demonstrate high content validity.[18,19,84–87] Different sources are used to generate an exhaustive list of all the relevant HRQOL issues: a systematically based literature review, interviews with patients, and interviews with health care professionals (HCPs). A vital and direct source of HRQOL issues is in-depth patient interviews or focus groups, which should be undertaken with a representative sample of the intended population. Typically, 20 to 30 patient interviews are required.

The provisional list of items generated by the literature review and patient interviews is then presented to a new, smaller sample of patients and HCPs to check for any ambiguities and missing items and for the relevance and importance of the identified items. If the HRQOL assessment tool is designed to be used in different countries (eg, as part of an international multicenter clinical trial), rigorous attention should be paid to the translation of HRQOL assessment.[84]

Phase 2: construction of the item list

Once the list of relevant HRQOL items is complete, it needs to be converted into questions. It is important to standardize the format of the questions and preferable to ask about the same time frame (eg, "during the past week"). It is also important to ensure that questions are clear, brief, and unambiguous; they should ask for only one piece of information. For example, "Do you feel weak and tired?" should be rephrased as 2 questions: "Do you feel weak?" and "Do you feel tired?" If there are several items covering similar constructs, they can be grouped in a hypothesized scale structure.

The resulting provisional list of items is then checked for clarity and overlap by a small number of patients from the target population who have not been previously interviewed and by a new group of HCPs.

Phase 3: pretesting the HRQOL assessment tool

The aim of pretesting the HRQOL assessment tool is to identify and solve potential problems in its administration and to identify missing or redundant issues. Patients from the target population who have not previously taken part in the development process are asked to complete the questionnaire and rate the importance and relevance of each item. A structured interview is then conducted with each patient to ensure completeness and acceptability of the items in the list. It is important to ensure that patients adequately represent the target population for which the questionnaire is being devised, so it is advisable to draw up a sample matrix to include all the relevant treatments and patient groups and to ensure patients are recruited to all cells in the matrix.

Based on this pretesting phase, the provisional questionnaire may require some adaptation (eg, changes to wording). In addition, it is important to consider whether each individual item should be retained or rejected, based on the information provided by the patients. To minimize respondent burden, it is important to retain only those items that are essential.

Phase 4: field testing

The final stage of development is field testing the questionnaire in a large, representative group of patients to determine its acceptability, reliability, validity, responsiveness, and cross-cultural applicability, as outlined in **Table 2**. The actual sample size required will depend on the number of items, the number of scales, the magnitude of the correlations, and the heterogeneity of the sample, but it is likely to be a few hundred. After completing the questionnaire, patients are asked to fill out a de-briefing questionnaire to check the length of time needed to complete the questionnaire, the amount and type of assistance required (if any), and whether any of the questions were confusing or upsetting. The debriefing questionnaire is used to determine the acceptability of the questionnaire. Both the internal reliability of the questionnaire and the test-retest reliability should be assessed. The internal reliability is a measure of whether the questionnaire's hypothesized scale structure is reliable. Test-retest reliability is checked by asking clinically stable patients to repeat the questionnaire 1 or 2 weeks after the first questionnaire. The external validity of the questionnaire can be assessed by comparing the results of the questionnaire with additional information collected at the same time. Responsiveness is addressed by comparing the results of questionnaires filled out at 2 time points by patients who experience a clinical change. At the end of phase 4, there may be a final reduction in the number of items in the questionnaire following psychometric analysis. A report on the development and validation of the HRQOL assessment tool should be published.

Use of HRQOL assessment in surgical decision making

An important question for the surgical team concerns how useful HRQOL assessment tools are in decision making. Their uses as a screening tool, aiding the monitoring of disease and treatment response, improving communication between clinician and patient, and improving quality of care, are all highlighted in the literature.[88–90]

Although there has been a lack of evidence to support the use of HRQOL assessments in clinical practice, this is a growing area of investigation. A systematic review[91] identified 23 trials that had examined the value of patient-reported outcome information to HCPs in daily clinical practice, with 15 studies identifying a significant effect in improving the process of care (eg, communication) and with 8 studies demonstrating improved outcomes (eg, improved functional status, HRQOL, and satisfaction with care). Although there are promising results from some trials, there were several

methodologic concerns that limited the review's conclusions; varying impact was demonstrated, and the review concluded that there was a need for greater clarity on the most important benefits that PROMs may yield when used in this way.

A trial has examined the use of preference-based HRQOL measures in routine clinical care of lung transplantation patients[92,93]; 231 patients were randomly assigned to 1 of 2 groups. Both groups completed the Health Utilities Index on touch-screen computers, but one group had feedback from clinicians and the other group completed the Health Utilities Index without feedback. All patients completed the EQ-5D as the HRQOL outcome at the end of the consultation. No significant difference in EQ-5D was demonstrated, with the authors claiming small effects on communication and small effects in patient management and HRQOL. However, several limitations (including the use of generic preference-based measures) need to be acknowledged. A summary of specific considerations for the use of HRQOL assessment tools in routine surgical patient management is outlined in **Box 1**.

AREAS FOR FUTURE CONSIDERATION
Use of Modern Psychometric Approaches

The emergence of modern measurement approaches may offer substantial prospects to enhance the rigor and efficiency of PROMs.[7] For example, differential item functioning allows testing of whether one group responds differently to an item compared with another group, even when known differences are controlled for, thus allowing another approach to enhance the validity of an assessment tool if problem items are removed or revised.[82]

Development of symptom-based measures

The move toward PROMs allows the surgeon to adopt a range of measures that are most applicable to evaluate the benefits of surgery. For some studies, the expected endpoint may be symptom improvement,[94,95] instead of HRQOL. There is a definite requirement for PROMs to respond quickly to new technologies, without compromise of quality. One of the main advances has been the construction of item banks[96,97] from well-established assessment tools. These item banks contain a range of HRQOL items (and responses), which can be drawn on to adapt or create new HRQOL assessment tools (eg, through computer adaptive testing).[98] The authors are undertaking an international project to develop scientifically robust, time-efficient procedures for the development of symptom-based measures

> **Box 1**
> **Considerations for the use of HRQOL assessment tools in management of pulmonary surgical patients**
>
> - Is the HRQOL assessment sufficiently responsive to patient response to surgery?
> - Can the collection of HRQOL data be timed appropriately to capture the greatest HRQOL changes?
> - Can the HRQOL assessment tool be used along other assessments as part of "patient-centered assessment"?
> - Is the HRQOL assessment able to give real-time results that can be easily interpreted by the surgical team and patient?
> - Can HRQOL assessment be incorporated into clinical training and education so surgical teams know how to use and interpret it?
> - Is the HRQOL assessment tool able to give clear information on what constitutes a clinically important change for the patient?
> - Is the HRQOL tool suitable for use across all patient demographics (eg, if using information technology, the ability of patients to complete using this method needs to be considered)?
> - Can HRQOL data collection be completed at regular follow-up?
> - Are the time and resources available to support HRQOL assessment?

for use in clinical trials and studies and will be providing guidelines that will be transferable to thoracic surgical populations.

HRQOL assessment as part of selecting patients for pulmonary surgery

There have been proposals for the use of risk assessment in the selection of patients with lung cancer to undergo surgery,[15] stressing the importance of clinical parameters and performance status. However, HRQOL receives little consideration even though many surgeons accept the importance of improving QOL as one of the most important considerations when deciding on surgery. The authors stress the potential for including a standardized HRQOL assessment in any comprehensive assessment of selecting patients for surgery, and further exploration is needed.

HRQOL in the evaluation of the quality of surgical care

Within the UK National Health Service, it has been recommended that PROMs should have a greater role.[99] In England, patient-reported outcomes are

routinely collected as part of a pilot initiative in some National Health Service surgical populations, including varicose vein, hip and knee replacement, and groin hernia surgery.[100] In a few years, HRQOL assessment could become commonplace in health care organizations.

SUMMARY

There is a requirement for careful attention to be paid when choosing, using, and developing HRQOL assessment tools in pulmonary surgery populations. There is increasing evidence to support the use of HRQOL assessment, with moves to using standard approaches. However, some limitations remain, as exemplified with recent studies of HRQOL in lung cancer surgical populations. New developments in patient-reported outcome measurement are showing potential in providing ways for the surgical team to ensure that HRQOL assessment provides clinically meaningful, robust information that places the patient perspective at the center of surgical decision making.

REFERENCES

1. Bowling A. Measuring disease. 2nd edition. Buckingham (England): Open University Press; 2001.
2. Rapley M. Quality of life research. London: Sage Publication; 2003.
3. Aaronson NK. Quality of life research in cancer clinical trials: a need for common rules and language. Oncology 1990;4:59–66.
4. Darzi A. High quality care for all: NHS next stage review final report. London: The Stationary Office; 2008. Available at: http://www.dh.gov.uk/prod_consum_dh/groups/dh_digitalassets/@dh/@en/documents/digitalasset/dh_085828.pdf. Accessed April 17, 2012.
5. Avery K, Blazeby JM. Quality of life assessment in surgical oncology trials. World J Surg 2006;30:1163–72.
6. Avery KN, Gujral S, Blazeby JM. Patient-reported outcomes to evaluate surgery. Expert Rev Pharmacoecon Outcomes Res 2008;8:43–50.
7. Kind P, Lafata JE, Matuszewski K, et al. The use of QALYs in clinical and patient decision-making: issues and prospects. Value Health 2009;12:S27–30.
8. Lipscomb J, Gotay CC, Snyder CF. Patient-reported outcomes in cancer: a review of recent research and policy initiatives. CA Cancer J Clin 2007;57:278–300.
9. US Food and Drug Administration. Guidance for industry patient-reported outcome measures: use in medical product development to support labelling claims. 2009. Available at: http://www.ispor.org/workpaper/FDA%20PRO%20Guidance.pdf. Accessed April 17, 2012.

10. Balducyck B, Hendriks J, Sardari NP, et al. Quality of life after lung cancer surgery: a review. Minerva Chir 2009;64:655–63.

11. Hahn EA, Cella D, Chassany O, et al. Precision of health-related quality of life data compared with other clinical measures. Mayo Clin Proc 2007;82: 1244–54.

12. Davis K, Yount S, Wagner L, et al. Measurement and management of health-related quality of life in lung cancer. Clin Adv Hematol Oncol 2004;2:533–40.

13. Yusen RD. Technology and outcomes assessment in lung transplantation. Proc Am Thorac Soc 2009;6:128–36.

14. Blazeby JM, Avery K, Sprangers M, et al. Health-related quality of life in randomised clinical trials in surgical oncology. J Clin Oncol 2006;24: 3178–86.

15. Brunelli A. Risk assessment for pulmonary resection. Semin Thorac Cardiovasc Surg 2010;22: 2–13.

16. Parasmeswaran R, McNair A, Avery KNL, et al. The role of health-related quality of life outcomes in clinical decision making in surgery for esophageal cancer: a systematic review. Ann Surg Oncol 2008;15:2372–9.

17. Karanicolas PJ, Bickenbash K, Jayaraman S, et al. Measurement and interpretation of patient-reported outcomes in surgery: an opportunity for improvement. J Gastrointest Surg 2011;15:682–9.

18. Patrick DL, Burke LB, Powers JH, et al. Patient reported outcomes to support medical product labelling claims: FDA perspective. Value Health 2007; 10:S125–37.

19. Rothman ML, Beltran P, Cappelleri JC, et al. Patient-reported outcomes: conceptual issues. Value Health 2007;10:S66–75.

20. Whitehead SJ, Ali S. Health outcomes in economic evaluation: the QALY and utilities. Br Med Bull 2010;96:5–21.

21. Brazier J, Ratcliffe J, Tshuiya A, et al. Measuring and valuing health benefits for economic evaluation. Oxford (United Kingdom): Oxford University Press; 2007.

22. EUROQOL Group. What is the EQ-5D? Available at: http://www.euroqol.org/home.html. Accessed April 17, 2012.

23. Brazier J, Roberts J, Deverill M. The estimation of a preference-based measure of health from the SF-36. J Health Econ 2002;21:271–92.

24. Yang Y, Brazier JE, Tsuchiya A, et al. Estimating a preference-based index for a 5 dimensional health state classification for asthma derived from the asthma quality of life questionnaire. Med Decis Making 2011;31:281–91.

25. Rowen D, Brazier J, Young T, et al. Developing a preference-based measure for cancer using the EORTC QLQ-C30. Value Health 2011;14:721–31.

26. Ware JE, Sherbourne CD. The MOS 36-item Short Form Survey (SF-36). Conceptual framework and item selection. Med Care 1992;30:473–83.

27. Streiner DL, Norman GR. Health measurement scales. A practical guide to their development and use. 4th edition. Oxford (United Kingdom): Oxford University Press; 2008.

28. Fitzpatrick R, Davey C, Buxton M. Evaluating patient-based outcome measures for use in clinical trials. Health Technol Assess 1998;2(14):i–iv, 1–74.

29. Efficace F, Bottomley A, Osoba D, et al. Beyond the development of health-related quality-of-life (HRQOL) measures: a checklist for evaluating HRQOL outcomes in cancer clinical trials: does HRQOL evaluation in prostate cancer research inform clinical decision making? J Clin Oncol 2003;21:3502–11.

30. Mokkink LB, Terwee CB, Patrick DL, et al. The COSMIN study reached international consensus on taxonomy, terminology and definitions of measurement properties for health-related patient-reported outcomes. J Clin Epidemiol 2010;63:737–45.

31. Zigmond AS, Snaith RP. The Hospital Anxiety and Depression Scale. Acta Psychiatr Scand 1983;67: 361–70.

32. Jones PW, Quirk FH, Baveystock CM, et al. A self-complete measure of health status for chronic airflow limitation. Am Rev Respir Dis 1992;45:1321–7.

33. Guyatt GH, Berman LB, Townsend M, et al. A measure of quality of life for clinical trials in chronic lung disease. Thorax 1987;42:773–8.

34. Cella DF, Bonomi AE, Lloyd SR, et al. Reliability and validity of the Functional Assessment of Cancer Therapy-Lung (FACT-L) quality of life instrument. Lung Cancer 1995;12:199–220.

35. Bergman B, Aaronson NK, Ahmedzai S, et al. The EORTC QLQ-LC13: a modular supplement to the EORTC quality of life questionnaire (QLQ-C3) for use in lung cancer clinical trials. EORTC Study Group on Quality of Life. Eur J Cancer 1994;30A: 635–42.

36. Juniper EF. Validated questionnaires should not be modified. Eur Respir J 2009;34:1015–7.

37. Benzo R, Farrell MH, Chang CC, et al, NETT Research Group. Integrating health status and survival data: the palliative effect of lung volume reduction surgery. Am J Respir Crit Care Med 2009;180:239–46.

38. Balduyck B, Hendriks J, Lauwers P, et al. Quality of life evolution after surgery for primary or secondary spontaneous pneumothorax: a prospective study comparing different surgical techniques. Interact Cardiovasc Thorac Surg 2008;7:45–9.

39. Rodrigue JR, Baz MA. Are there sex differences in health-related quality of life after lung transplantation for chronic obstructive pulmonary disease? J Heart Lung Transplant 2006;25:120–5.

40. Chen H, Taichman DB, Doyle RL. Health-related quality of life and patient-reported outcomes in pulmonary arterial hypertension. Proc Am Thorac Soc 2008;15:623–30.

41. De Vries J, Drent M. Quality of life and health status in interstitial lung diseases. Curr Opin Pulm Med 2006;12:354–8.

42. Swigris JJ, Kushner WG, Jacobs SS, et al. Health-related quality of life in patients with idiopathic pulmonary fibrosis: a systematic review. Thorax 2005;60:588–94.

43. Doll H, Miravitlies M. Health-related QOL in acute exacerbations of chronic bronchitis and chronic obstructive pulmonary disease: a review of the literature. Pharmacoeconomics 2005;23:345–63.

44. Bottomley A, Efficace F, Thomas R, et al. Health-related quality of life in non-small-cell lung cancer: methodological issues in randomised controlled trials. J Clin Oncol 2003;21:2982–92.

45. Handy JR. Functional outcomes after lung cancer resection. Who cares as long as you are cured? Chest 2009;135:258–9.

46. Classens L, van Meerbeeck J, Coens C, et al. Health-related quality of life in non-small-cell lung cancer: an update of a systematic review on methodological issues in randomised controlled trials. J Clin Oncol 2011;29:2104–20.

47. Fitzsimmons D, Gilbert J, Howse F, et al. A systematic review of the use and validation of health-related quality of life instruments in older cancer patients. Eur J Cancer 2009;45:19–32.

48. Balduyck B, Hendriks J, Lauwers P, et al. Quality of life evolution after lung cancer surgery: a prospective study in 100 patients. Lung Cancer 2007;56(3):423–31.

49. Balduyck B, Hendriks J, Lauwers P, et al. Quality of life after lung cancer surgery: a prospective pilot study comparing bronchial sleeve lobectomy with pneumonectomy. J Thorac Oncol 2008;3:604–8.

50. Balduyck B, Hendriks J, Lauwers P, et al. Quality of life evolution after lung surgery in septuagenarians: a prospective study. Eur J Cardiothorac Surg 2009;35:1070–5.

51. Kenney PM, King MT, Viney RC, et al. Quality of life and survival in the 2 years after surgery for non-small-cell lung cancer. J Clin Oncol 2008;26:233–41.

52. Schulte T, Schniewind B, Dohrmann P, et al. The extent of lung parenchyma resection significantly impacts long-term quality of life in patients with non-small cell lung cancer. Chest 2009;13:322–9.

53. Schulte T, Schniewind B, Dohrmann P, et al. Age-related impairment of quality of life after lung resection for non-small cell lung cancer. Lung Cancer 2010;68:115–20.

54. Win T, Sharples L, Wells FC, et al. Effect of lung cancer surgery on quality of life. Thorax 2005;60:234–8.

55. Brunelli A, Socci L, Refai M, et al. Quality of life before and after major lung resection for lung cancer: a prospective follow-up analysis. Ann Thorac Surg 2007;84:410–6.

56. Handy JR Jr, Asaph JW, Douville EC, et al. Does video-assisted thorascopic lobectomy for lung cancer provide improved functional outcomes compared with open lobectomy? Eur J Cardiothorac Surg 2010;32(2):451–5.

57. Heuker D, Lengele B, Delecluse V, et al. Subjective and objective assessment of quality of life after chest wall resection. Eur J Cardiothorac Surg 2011;39(1):102–8.

58. Moller A, Sartiby U. Changes in quality of life after lung surgery in old and young patients: are they similar? World J Surg 2010;34:684–91.

59. Moller A, Sartiby U. Long term health-related quality of life following surgery for lung cancer. Eur J Cardiothorac Surg 2012;41:362–7.

60. Pompili C, Brunelli A, Xiume F, et al. Predictors of postoperative decline in quality of life after major lung resection. Eur J Cardiothorac Surg 2011;39:732–7.

61. Sarna L, Cooly ME, Brown JK, et al. Women with lung cancer: quality of life after thoracotomy. Cancer Nurs 2010;33:85–92.

62. Salati M, Brunelli S, Xiume F, et al. Quality of life in the elderly after major lung resection of lung cancer. Interact Cardiovasc Thorac Surg 2009;8:79–83.

63. Sartipy U. Prospective population-based study comparing quality of life after pneumonectomy and lobectomy. Eur J Cardiothorac Surg 2009;36:1069–74.

64. Sartipy U. Influence of gender on quality of life after lung cancer. Eur J Cardiothorac Surg 2010;37:802–6.

65. Ilonen IK, Rasanen JV, Knuuttila A, et al. Quality of life following lobectomy or bilobectomy for non-small-cell lung cancer: a two year prospective study. Lung Cancer 2010;70:347–51.

66. Pompili C, Brunelli A, Xiume F, et al. Prospective external convergence evaluation of two different quality-of-life instruments in lung resection patients. Eur J Cardiothorac Surg 2011;4:99–105.

67. Li WW, Lee TW, Yim AP. Quality of life after lung cancer resection. Thorac Surg Clin 2004;14:353–65.

68. Berger RL, Wood KA, Cabral HJ, et al. Lung volume reduction surgery: a meta-analysis of randomized clinical trials. Treat Respir Med 2005;4:201–9.

69. I Comabella CC, Gibbons E, Fitzpatrick R. A structured review of patient-reported outcome measures for patients with lung cancer. Report to the Department of Health; 2010. Available at: http://phi.uhce.ox.ac.uk/pdf/CancerReviews/PROMs_Oxford_Lung%20Cancer_012011.pdf. Accessed April 20, 2012.

70. Williamson P, Altman D, Blazeby J, et al. Driving up the quality of relevance of research through the use

of agreed core outcomes. J Health Serv Res Policy 2012;17:1–2.

71. Calvert M, Blazeby J, Revicki D, et al. Reporting quality of life in clinical trials: a consort extension. Lancet 2011;378:1684–5.

72. Schwartz CE, Bode R, Repucci N, et al. The clinical significance of adaptation to changing health: a meta-analysis of response shift. Qual Life Res 2006;15:1533–50.

73. Yun YH, Kim YA, Min YH, et al. Health-related quality of life in disease-free survivors of surgically treated lung cancer compared with the general population. Ann Surg 2012;255:1000–7.

74. Sugimura H, Yang P. Long-term survivorship in lung cancer: a review. Chest 2006;129:1088–97.

75. Revicki D, Hays RD, Cella D, et al. Recommended methods for determining responsiveness and minimally important differences for patient-reported outcomes. J Clin Epidemiol 2006;61:102–9.

76. Land SR. Missing patient-reported outcome data in an adjuvant lung cancer study. J Clin Oncol 2008; 26:5018–9.

77. Gonzalez-Aragoneses F, Moreno-Mata N, Simon-Adigo C, et al. Lung cancer surgery in the elderly. Crit Rev Oncol Hematol 2009;71:266–71.

78. Chambers A, Routledge T, Pilling J, et al. In elderly patients with lung cancer is resection in terms of morbidity, mortality and residual quality of life? Interact Cardiovasc Thorac Surg 2010;10:1015–21.

79. Johnson C, Fitzsimmons D, Gilbert J, et al, EORTC Quality of Life Group. Development of the european organisation for research and treatment of cancer quality of life questionnaire module for older people with cancer: the EORTC QLQ-ELD15. Eur J Cancer 2010;46:2242–52.

80. European Medicines Agency, Committee for Medicinal Products for Human Use (CHMP). Reflection paper on the regulatory guidance for the use of health-related quality of life (HRQL) measures in the evaluation of medicinal products. 2005. Available at: http://www.ispor.org/workpaper/emea-hrql-guidance.pdf. Accessed April 20, 2012.

81. Synder CF, Watson ME, Jackson JD, et al, Mayo/FDA Patient-Reported Outcomes Consensus Meeting Group. Patient-reported outcome instrument selection: designing a measurement strategy. Value Health 2007;10:S76–85.

82. Frost MH, Reeve BB, Liepa AM, et al, Mayo/FDA Patient-reported Outcomes Consensus Meeting Group. What is sufficient evidence for the reliability and validity of patient-reported outcome measures? Value Health 2007;10:S94–105.

83. Johnson C, Aaronson N, Blazeby JM, et al. EORTC Quality of Life Group Guidelines for DevelopingQuestionnaire Modules. 4th edition. Brussels (Belgium): EORTC QL Group; 2011. Available at: http://groups. eortc.be/qol/Pdf%20presentations/Guidelines%20

for%20Developing%20questionnaire-%20FINAL.pdf. Accessed April 20, 2012.

84. Rothman M, Burke L, Erickson P, et al. Use of existing patient-reported outcome (PRO) instruments and their modification: the ISPOR good research practices for evaluating and documenting content validity for the use of existing instruments and their modification PRO task force report. Value Health 2009;12:1075–103.

85. Dewolf L, Koller M, Velikova G, et al, EORTC Quality of Life Group. EORTC quality of life group translation procedure. Brussels (Belgium): EORTC; 2009. Available at: http://groups.eortc.be/qol/downloads/translation_manual_2009.pdf. Accessed April 20, 2012.

86. Guyatt G, Schunemann H. How can quality of life researchers make their work more useful to health workers and their patients? Qual Life Res 2007; 16:1097–105.

87. King MT, Fayers PM. Making quality-of-life results more meaningful for clinicians. Lancet 2008;371: 709–10.

88. Lohr KN, Zebrack BJ. Using patient-reported outcomes in clinical practice: challenges and opportunities. Qual Life Res 2009;18:99–107.

89. Fung CH, Hays RD. Prospects and challenges in using patient-reported outcomes in clinical practice. Qual Life Res 2008;17:1297–302.

90. Osoba D. What has been learned from measuring health-related quality of life in clinical oncology? Eur J Cancer 1999;35(11):1565–70.

91. Valderas JM, Kotzeva A, Esparallargues M, et al. The impact of measuring patient-reported outcomes in clinical practice: a systematic review of the literature. Qual Life Res 2008;17:179–93.

92. Santana MJ, Feeny D, Johnson JA, et al. Assessing the use of health-related quality of life measures in the routine clinical care of lung-transplant patients. Qual Life Res 2010;19:371–9.

93. Semik M, Schmid C, Trosch F, et al. Lung cancer surgery-preoperative risk assessment and patient selection. Lung Cancer 2001;33(Suppl 1):$9–$15.

94. Osoba D. Translating the science of patient-reported outcomes into clinical practice. J Natl Cancer Inst Monogr 2007;37:5–11.

95. Cleeland CS, Sloan JA. Assessing the symptoms of cancer using patient-reported outcomes (ASPRCO): searching for standards. J Pain Symptom Manage 2010;39:1077–85.

96. Revicki DA, Sloan J. Practical and philosophical issues surrounding a national item bank: if we build it will they come? Qual Life Res 2007;16:167–74.

97. Vachalec S, Bjordal K, Bottomley A, et al, EORTC Quality of Life Group. EORTC item bank guidelines. Brussels (Belgium): EORTC; 2010. Available at: http://groups.eortc.be/qol/downloads/200104item bank_guidelines.pdf. Accessed April 20, 2012.

98. Peterson MA, Groenvold M, Aaronson N, et al,
European Organisation for Research and Treatment of Cancer Quality of Life Group. Multidimensional computerised adaptive testing of the
EORTC QLQ-C30: basic developments and evaluations. Qual Life Res 2006;15:315–29.

99. Devlin NJ, Appleby J. Getting the most out of
PROMS putting health outcomes at the heart of
NHS decision-making. London: Kings Fund;
2010. Available at: http://www.kingsfund.org.uk/
publications/proms.html. Accessed April 20,
2012.

100. Department of Health. Guidance on the routine
collection of patient reported outcome measures
(PROMs). London: Department of Health; 2008.
Available at: http://www.dh.gov.uk/en/Publications
andstatistics/Publications/PublicationsPolicyAnd
Guidance/DH_092647. Accessed April 20, 2012.

Changes in Quality of Life After Pulmonary Resection

Alessandro Brunelli, MD[a],*, Cecilia Pompili, MD[b], Michael Koller, PhD[c]

KEYWORDS

- Quality of life • Pulmonary resection • Lung cancer • Postoperative course

KEY POINTS

- In this study pulmonary lobectomy had a transient influence on physical functioning with subsequent partial recovery over time, but no other quality-of-life scales were affected.
- Pneumonectomy had a large impact on physical and emotional domains. These quality-of-life scales did not show any recovery during follow-up, and many of them declined even more over time.
- Every effort should be made to avoid pneumonectomy whenever technically and oncologically feasible.

INTRODUCTION

Patient-centered outcomes have become an important aspect of perioperative evaluations. A patient's fears, expectations, and judgment should be taken into account when selecting the most appropriate treatment for that person.

Most recent guidelines have emphasized the central role of the patient in accepting or refusing surgical risks based on expected postoperative quality of life (QoL).[1] On the other hand, the prediction of postoperative QoL, which is a subjective measure, by means of objective parameters that are commonly used to estimate surgical risks (ie, pulmonary function tests, diffusion capacity of lung for carbon monoxide [DLCO], age, and so forth) has been proved to be inaccurate.[2–4] Furthermore, the effect of pulmonary surgery on QoL has been investigated in a growing number of trials in recent years; however, the instruments and metrics used for analysis have varied, which complicates the interpretation and generalization of such trials.[5]

A synthesis of the available data comparing preoperative and postoperative QoL after lung resection may assist physicians during surgical counseling. The objective of this study was to assess the impact of pulmonary resection on QoL by means of a systematic, quantitative review of the available literature.

METHODOLOGY

Eligibility Criteria

The following trials were eligible for inclusion: randomized, nonrandomized, and retrospective trials on patients who had undergone surgery for lung cancer and had been assessed preoperatively and postoperatively with regard to QoL measures.

Information Sources

Trials were identified by searching electronic databases (PubMed and Google Scholar) and

The authors have nothing to disclose.
[a] Section of Minimally Invasive Thoracic Surgery, Division of Thoracic Surgery, Ospedali Riuniti Ancona, Via Conca 1, 60122 Ancona, Italy; [b] Division of Thoracic Surgery, Ospedali Riuniti Ancona, Via Conca 1, 60122 Ancona, Italy; [c] Center for Clinical Studies, University Hospital Regensburg, 93042 Regensburg, Germany
* Corresponding author. Division of Thoracic Surgery, Ospedali Riuniti Ancona, Via Conca 1, 60122 Ancona, Italy.
E-mail address: brunellialex@gmail.com

Thorac Surg Clin 22 (2012) 471–485
http://dx.doi.org/10.1016/j.thorsurg.2012.07.006
1547-4127/12/$ – see front matter © 2012 Elsevier Inc. All rights reserved

examining references of relevant publications. PubMed was searched for English-language articles meeting the eligibility criteria and published between January 1, 2000, and March 2012.

References of relevant articles and book chapters were also searched.

Search

To assist the electronic evidence search, the following PICO (Patient, Intervention, Control, Outcome) question strategy was developed: "What is the residual QoL of patients with lung cancer submitted to pulmonary resection compared with preoperative status?" The following key words were used for the PubMed search: (nonsmall cell lung cancer) AND (quality of life) AND (resection or surgery). Restrictions included dates (1/1/2000 to 03/01/2012), English language, and trials in humans.

Study Selection

Eligibility was independently assessed by 2 separate authors in an unblinded, standardized manner by screening titles and abstracts identified by the previously described searches and sources. Disagreements between reviewers were resolved by consensus. The full texts of selected trials were reviewed and assessed further.

Data-Collection Process

Data from eligible studies were extracted by one author and then independently by a second author. A table of evidence was created (**Table 1**). Disagreements were solved by discussions between the 2 authors. The authors of 5 of the trials[6,8,9,14,16] included in the systematic review were contacted to obtain sufficient data for the quantitative analysis. Unpublished data were received from these investigators.

Data Items

Variables for which data were sought included patient-related information (number of patients overall and in each group, age, and so forth), the inclusion and exclusion criteria of a trial, the type of intervention (lobectomy, pneumonectomy), the type of surgical access (thoracotomy, video-assisted thoracoscopic surgery [VATS]), the instruments and metrics used to assess QoL (Short Form 36 [SF36], European Organization for the Research and Treatment of Cancer [EORTC] C30, LC13 QoL surveys, and so forth), the preoperative QoL, the postoperative QoL measures, and the timing of the postoperative assessment.

Synthesis of Data

Perioperative changes in the QoL scales were measured by means of the Cohen effect-size method (mean change of the variable divided by its baseline standard deviation).[19] An effect size of >0.8 (or <-0.8) is regarded as large and clinically relevant, whereas an effect size between 0.3 and 0.8 or lower than 0.3 is regarded as medium or small, respectively.[20] To provide a summary measure for each QoL dimension, mean effect sizes of the same concept scales from different QoL instruments were calculated (ie, SF36 social functioning and EORTC social functioning, SF36 physical functioning and EORTC physical functioning, SF36 RP−role limitation caused by physical problems and EORTC RF−role functioning, SF36 RE−role limitation caused by emotional problems and EORTC EF−emotional functioning, SF36 MH−mental health and EORTC CF−cognitive functioning, SF36 GH-general health perception and EORTC GHS−global health scale). Data from the same investigators' groups exploring different aspects of a subject but partially or completely including the same patients were synthesized in a single analysis without any duplication. For instance, the data of different articles published by the Ancona group were updated and merged, and generated one single unified analysis.

RESULTS OF QUANTITATIVE ANALYSIS

A total of 15 trials met the inclusion criteria. No randomized trial was found.

Nine trials used the SF36 and 6 the EORTC C30 as an instrument to measure QoL.

Table 1 summarizes the main findings of these studies.

Table 2 shows the standardized mean perioperative differences (effect size) of patients after lobectomy derived from trials assessing postoperative QoL at 3 months. Only one trial[14] showed a large reduction in the physical functioning domain after lobectomy at 3 months.

Table 3 shows the standardized mean perioperative differences (effect size) of patients after lobectomy derived from trials assessing postoperative QoL at 6 months. Only one study[14] showed a large reduction in the physical functioning domain after lobectomy at 6 months.

Table 4 shows the standardized mean perioperative differences (effect size) of patients after lobectomy derived from trials assessing postoperative QoL at greater than 6 months. Schulte and colleagues[14] confirmed a large reduction of physical functioning (PF) at 12 months after lobectomy.

Table 1
Table of evidence summarizing the findings of all trials reporting perioperative measurements of QoL scales

Authors[Ref.]	Year	No. of Patients	Groups Compared	Assessment Instrument	Time of Assessment	Major Findings Quantitatively	Major Findings Summarized in Words
Balduyck et al[6]	2007	100	Patients with major pulmonary resection for cancer	EORTC Q30 + LC13	Preoperatively, 1, 3, 6, and 12 mo postoperatively	Both resections are characterized by a 1-mo temporary decrease in QoL functioning scores and an increase in pain symptoms After lobectomy, patients report an increase in dyspnea in the first postoperative month, not seen after wedge resection After pneumonectomy, values for physical functioning, role functioning, pain, shoulder function, and dyspnea do not return to baseline during a 12-mo follow-up period	After lobectomy, patients have more favorable physical functioning and less thoracic pain than patients after pneumonectomy Antero- and posterolateral thoracotomy are comparable for QoL evaluation
Brunelli et al[3]	2007	156	Patients with lobectomy and pneumonectomy for cancer	SF36	Preoperatively, 1 mo and 3 mo postoperatively	PCS was significantly reduced at 1 mo (51 vs 45.1, $P<.0001$), and completely recovered at 3 mo (51 vs 52.4, $P = .2$), whereas MCS remained unchanged No difference in high-risk patients. No correlation with functional variables	Patients for lung resection for lung cancer had worse preoperative QoL than the general population The functional variables cannot substitute for specific evaluation instruments
Burfeind et al[7]	2008	422	Patients with lobectomy group 1 ≤70 y and group 2 ≥70 y	EORTC QLQ-C30 + LC13	Preoperatively, 3, 6, and 12 mo postoperatively	Postoperative decrease in QoL at 3 mo At 6 and 12 mo, all domains had returned to baseline except PF, which remained below baseline in group 2. EF improved postoperatively for both groups	Quality of life outcomes are equivalent after lobectomy in older and younger patients

(continued on next page)

Table 1
(continued)

Authors[Ref.]	Year	No. of Patients	Groups Compared	Assessment Instrument	Time of Assessment	Major Findings Quantitatively	Major Findings Summarized in Words
Handy et al[8]	2002	103	Patients after lung cancer surgery	SF36 + QLI	Preoperatively and 6 mo postoperatively	Preoperatively worse results on the SF36 PF, RE, MH, E subscales At 6 mo, SF36 subscales for PF, RF, RP, BP, and MH were significantly worse than preoperative values. Low preoperative DLCO predicted poor postoperative QLI	Pain and impairment of functional health status persists for 6 mo after lung cancer resection. DLCO, not FEV$_1$, predicts postoperative QoL
Handy et al[9]	2010	241	Lung cancer lobectomy OPEN group vs VATS group	SF36 + QLI	Preoperatively and 6 mo postoperatively	VATS patients had either the same or better values in all SF36 categories The OPEN group, however, had significantly worse values in SF36 PF, RF. Postoperative BP and GH were significantly improved over preoperative values in the VATS group No difference between preoperative and 6-mo postoperative VATS vs OPEN QLI scores	VATS lobectomy for curative lung cancer resection appears to provide superior functional health recovery compared with OPEN techniques
Moller and Sartipy[10]	2012	213	Surgical patients for lung cancer	SF36	Preoperatively and 6 mo postoperatively	The extent of resection and adjuvant therapy was significantly associated with a clinically relevant decline in the SF36 PCS	The extent of resection and adjuvant therapy was associated with a clinically relevant decline in the physical aspect of health-related QoL 6 mo after surgery

Leo et al[11]	2010	41	Pneumonectomy patients for lung cancer	EORTC QLQ-C30 + LC13	Preoperatively, 1, 3, 6 mo postoperatively	6 mo after pneumonectomy, global health showed minimal impairment in the whole population. Age of 70 y or more was identified as a significant risk factor for poor 6-mo QoL. The baseline global health score was the strongest predictor of postoperative global health QoL	The overall QoL after pneumonectomy was impaired in 25% of surviving patients at 6 mo after surgery
Pompili et al[12]	2010	220	Patients after lobectomy for lung cancer (COPD patients vs non-COPD patients)	SF36	Preoperatively and 3 mo postoperatively	No differences between the groups in any of the preoperative and postoperative physical and mental QoL scales	Evidence of an acceptable QoL in patients with COPD
Sartipy[13]	2009	117	Patients after lobectomy vs patients after pneumonectomy for lung cancer	SF36	Preoperatively and 6 mo postoperatively	Significant difference in the fractional change in the physical component summary score between the lobectomy and pneumonectomy group (-17% vs -32%, $P = .04$), but not in the mental component summary score (6.5% vs 12%, $P = .72$)	Pneumonectomy had a larger negative impact on the PCS than lobectomy 6 mo postoperatively. The MCS was not affected by the extent of surgical resection

(continued on next page)

Table 1
(continued)

Authors[Ref.]	Year	No. of Patients	Groups Compared	Assessment Instrument	Time of Assessment	Major Findings Quantitatively	Major Findings Summarized in Words
Schulte et al[14]	2009	159	Patients after lobectomy-bilobectomy vs patients after pneumonectomy for lung cancer	EORTC QLQ-C30 + LC13	Preoperatively and up to 24 mo postoperatively	After a postoperative drop, most QoL indicators remained near baseline for up to 24 mo, except for PF ($P<.001$), PAIN ($P = .034$), and dyspnea ($P<.001$), which remained significantly impaired QoL was significantly better after bilobectomy/lobectomy than after pneumonectomy Differences were significant with regards to PF (at 3 mo), SF (at 3 and 6 mo), RF (at 3, 6, and 12 mo), GH (at 3 and 6 mo), and pain (at 6 mo)	Patients who underwent lung resection for NSCLC failed to completely recover after 24 mo. Patients who underwent pneumonectomy had significantly worse QoL values and less tendency to recover
Schulte et al[15]	2009	131	Patients after lobectomy and patients after bilobectomy	EORTC QLQ-C30 + LC13	Preoperatively and up to 24 mo postoperatively	The QoL of younger patients returned to preoperative levels significantly faster than the QoL of elderly patients	Elderly patients had less tendency to achieve the preoperative level of QoL compared with younger ones
Kenny et al[16]	2008	173	Stage I–II resected NSCLC	EORTC QLQ-C30 + LC13	Preoperatively, at discharge, 1 mo after surgery, and then every 4 mo for 2 y	Surgery substantially reduced HR QoL across all dimensions except for EF. HR QoL improved in the 2 y after surgery for patients without disease recurrence. Patients with recurrence within 2 y sometimes recover early postoperatively in HR QoL, but subsequently deteriorate across most dimensions	HR QoL generally worsened after disease recurrence. Surgery had a substantial impact on HR QoL

Pompili et al[17]	2011	172	Patients after lobectomy and patients after pneumonectomy for lung cancer	SF36	Preoperatively and 3 mo postoperatively	28% of patients showed a large decline in the PCS scale and 15% in the MCS scale. Patients with better preoperative PF ($P = .0008$) and BP ($P = .048$) scores and those with worse MH ($P = .0007$) scores had a higher risk of relevant physical deterioration. Patients with a lower ppoFEV$_1$, higher preoperative scores of SF ($P = .02$) and MH ($P = .06$) had a higher risk of relevant emotional deterioration	A consistent proportion of patients undergoing lung resection exhibit important postoperative worsening in QoL. Predictive equations were developed to estimate the risk of decline in QoL
Salati et al[18]	2009	218	Patients after major lung resection (Group1: ≥70 y; Group2: <70 y)	SF36	Preoperatively and 3 mo postoperatively	Postoperative PCS and MCS did not differ between older and younger patients	QoL in the elderly is similar to that experienced by younger and fitter individuals

Abbreviations: BP, bodily pain; COPD, chronic obstructive pulmonary disease; DLCO, diffusion capacity of lung for carbon monoxide; E, emotion; EF, emotional-functioning subscale; EORTC, European Organization for the Research and Treatment of Cancer; FEV$_1$, predicted postoperative forced expiratory volume in 1 second; GH, global health subscale; HR, health-related; MCS, mental health composite scale; MH, mental health subscale; NSCLC, non–small cell lung cancer; PCS, physical composite scale; PF, physical-functioning subscale; ppoFEV$_1$, predicted postoperative FEV$_1$; QLI, Quality of Life Index; QLQ, Quality of Life Questionnaire; RE, role-limitation emotional subscale; RF, role-functioning subscale; RP, role-limitation physical subscale; SF36, Short Form 36; SF, social-functioning subscale; VATS, video-assisted thoracoscopic surgery.

Brunelli et al

Table 2
Standardized perioperative differences 3 months after lobectomy

Reference	Survey	No. of Patients	ES1	ES2	ES3	ES4	ES5	ES6
Ancona[3,12,17,18]	SF36	179	0.12	−0.35	−0.09	0.15	−0.03	−0.14
Balduyck et al[6]	EORTC	61	0.08	−0.30	−0.20	−0.32	0.44	−0.15
Burfeind et al[7]	EORTC	422	−0.29	−0.32	−0.41	−0.13	−0.03	−0.63
Schulte et al[14]	EORTC	127	−0.26	−0.98	−0.52	n.r.	n.r.	−0.77

An effect size of >0.8 (or <−0.8) is regarded as large, between 0.3 and 0.8 as medium, and <0.3 as small.
Abbreviations: ES1, SF36 GH—general health perception or EORTC GHS—global health scale; ES2, SF36 physical functioning or EORTC physical functioning; ES3, SF36 social functioning or EORTC social functioning; ES4, SF36 MH—mental health or EORTC CF—cognitive functioning; ES5, SF36 RE—role limitation caused by emotional problems or EORTC EF—emotional functioning; ES6, SF36 RP—role limitation caused by physical problems or EORTC RF—role functioning; n.r., not reported.

Five groups reported data on perioperative changes of QoL in patients after pneumonectomy. **Tables 5–7** show details of standardized perioperative differences at 3, 6, and 12 months after pneumonectomy. Most groups reported a large decline in the physical domains of QoL, which persisted up to 12 months after surgery.

Fig. 1 shows the average values of effect sizes at different postoperative times after pulmonary lobectomy. Most scales showed a trend of recovery from the first evaluation time point up to 12 months after surgery. PF was particularly depressed at 3 months and, despite its recovery, the change compared with its preoperative value remained at medium relevance at 6 and 12 months.

Fig. 2 shows the average values of effect sizes at different postoperative time points after pneumonectomy. Most scales showed a stable or declining trend from the first evaluation up to 12 months after surgery. PF and role limitation due to physical problems showed the largest decline and did not improve over time. In addition, emotional or mental domains also showed large negative changes compared with preoperative values.

SYNTHESIS OF EVIDENCE

Residual QoL after curative resection for lung cancer is a concept of increasing interest in both the medical literature and clinical practice. Residual QoL has become of crucial importance when informing patients about the risk of surgery and discussing the different treatment options with them.

One of the major concerns for patients is the possibility to resume an acceptable lifestyle. This factor has been reported to be even more important for patients than the fear of perioperative complications or mortality.[21]

Despite the increasing number of publications on this topic, the interpretation of the results is often difficult because of the different metrics, case mix, and evaluation times used. In addition, we still lack a reliable method for accurately estimating or predicting postoperative QoL, information which would be most valued by patients.

Table 3
Standardized perioperative differences 6 months after lobectomy

Reference	Survey	No. of Patients	ES1	ES2	ES3	ES4	ES5	ES6
Balduyck et al[6]	EORTC	61	0.25	−0.24	−0.04	0.12	0.21	−0.12
Burfeind et al[7]	EORTC	420	−0.44	−0.17	−0.13	−0.09	0.14	−0.24
Schulte et al[14]	EORTC	114	−0.17	−0.94	−0.35	n.r.	n.r.	−0.67
Handy et al,[8] 2002	SF36	103	−0.13	−0.37	−0.70	−0.29	−0.07	−0.20
Handy et al,[9] 2010 (thoracotomy)	SF36	100	−0.20	−0.54	−0.40	0.02	−0.25	−0.52
Handy et al,[9] 2010 (VATS)	SF36	25	0.24	−0.05	−0.08	0.23	−0.26	0.26
Sartipy,[13] 2009	SF36	101	−0.34	−0.43	0.0007	0.344	−0.12	−0.71

An effect size of >0.8 (or <−0.8) is regarded as large, between 0.3 and 0.8 as medium, and <0.3 as small.

Table 4
Standardized perioperative differences 12 months after lobectomy

Reference	Survey	No. of Patients	ES1	ES2	ES3	ES4	ES5	ES6
Balduyck et al[6]	EORTC	61	0.009	−0.290	0.030	−0.050	0.390	−0.060
Burfeind et al[7]	EORTC	403	0.030	−0.110	−0.070	−0.110	0.190	−0.100
Schulte et al[14]	EORTC	97	−0.090	−0.840	−0.440	n.r.	n.r.	−0.500
Kenny et al[16]	EORTC	87	0.120	−0.150	0	−0.160	0.430	−0.040

An effect size of >0.8 (or <−0.8) is regarded as large, between 0.3 and 0.8 as medium, and <0.3 as small.

In the attempt to standardize perioperative changes of QoL measures, the authors searched the available literature for preoperative and postoperative data on QoL and expressed the results as standardized mean differences regardless of the instruments used for their assessment (EORTC or SF36). In addition, information was broken down according to the extent of surgery (pneumonectomy vs lobectomy) and the follow-up period.

The extent of surgery has been consistently reported as the most important factor influencing QoL. Patients submitted to pneumonectomy report the most relevant decline in QoL, particularly in the physical domain. Moreover, time from surgery has been shown to be associated with QoL, with patients reporting the largest decline in QoL directly after surgery and experiencing a gradual recovery over time.

In the attempt to provide unified, clinically meaningful information, domains of different surveys (EORTC or SF36) related to similar concepts were grouped. Grouping was based on the conceptual meaning of each construct without evaluating the relative individual psychometric properties or their external convergence. This factor needs to be taken into consideration when interpreting the results presented here.

Three months after lobectomy, the scales related to social functioning (SF) and role limitation because of physical problems declined to medium relevance compared with preoperative values.

These scales gradually recovered in the following months. The most affected scale after lobectomy was PF, which showed a large decline in the first evaluation period (3 months after operation) compared with preoperative values. Although this scale showed recovery at 6 and 12 months, the standardized mean difference still remained at medium relevance.

Other scales more related to global health or emotional-status perception did not seem to be affected by lobectomy.

It was found that pneumonectomy had a more relevant impact than lobectomy on QoL. Although the number of patients who had undergone pneumonectomy and had been included in the few studies that separately analyzed the effect of this operation on QoL were relatively small (ranging from 14 to 41), negative effect sizes were generally larger than after lobectomy.

The fact that most scales remained stable or even worsened over time after pneumonectomy seems noteworthy. Only general health perception improved from medium to small negative change.

PF and role limitation because of physical problems showed an immediate large decline and did not improve over time, thus remaining stable or even worsening, respectively.

Emotional or mental domains showed negative changes of their standardized perioperative mean differences over time, of large (ES4) or medium (ES5) relevance at 12 months.

Table 5
Standardized perioperative differences 3 months after pneumonectomy

Reference	Survey	No. of Patients	ES1	ES2	ES3	ES4	ES5	ES6
Ancona[3,12,17,18]	SF36	14	−0.05	−0.26	−0.24	−0.04	0.15	−0.22
Balduyck et al[6]	EORTC	17	−0.39	−1.85	−0.42	−0.27	0.31	−2.65
Schulte et al[14]	EORTC	26	−0.54	−2.05	−0.80	n.r.	n.r.	−1.40

An effect size of >0.8 (or <−0.8) is regarded as large, between 0.3 and 0.8 as medium, and <0.3 as small.

Table 6
Standardized perioperative differences 6 months after pneumonectomy

Reference	Survey	No. of Patients	ES1	ES2	ES3	ES4	ES5	ES6
Balduyck et al[6]	EORTC	17	−0.04	−1.84	−0.46	−0.90	−0.10	−2.80
Schulte et al[14]	EORTC	21	−0.29	−1.80	−0.36	n.r.	n.r.	−1.14
Leo et al[11]	EORTC	41	−0.15	−0.20	−0.33	0.38	0.64	−0.11
Sartipy[13]	SF36	16	−0.82	−1.75	−0.44	0.07	−0.29	−0.83

An effect size of >0.8 (or <−0.8) is regarded as large, between 0.3 and 0.8 as medium, and <0.3 as small.

The SF domain remained stable during all postoperative evaluation times with an effect size of medium relevance.

Predictors of Postoperative Quality of Life

Pneumonectomy

The extent of this type of surgery has been consistently reported by many investigators as a factor that negatively affects residual QoL.[3,6,10,13,14,16]

Schulte and colleagues[14] reported that PF, SF, role functioning (RF), global health, and pain scales were significantly better (difference >10 points) after lobectomy than after pneumonectomy 3, 6, and 12 months after surgery.

Brunelli and colleagues[3] found that the physical component of QoL measured at 3 months after surgery was significantly lower after pneumonectomy than after lobectomy (−4.3 points).

Balduyck and colleagues[6] found that PF and RF were markedly and significantly reduced 3 months after pneumonectomy compared with preoperative values (−20 and −38.5, respectively). These changes remained stable at 6 months. Conversely, the same scales were minimally affected by lobectomy (−5.9 and −4.8, respectively).

Sartipy[13] reported a significant difference in the fractional change of the physical summary score between patients after lobectomy and patients after pneumonectomy (−17% vs −32%). The same group[10] found that the extent of resection had a significant impact on the physical component of QoL after surgery. However, in their trial the investigators pooled lobectomies and pneumonectomies and used sublobar resection as a reference.

The impact of pneumonectomy on the physical scales of perceived QoL is in line with the cardiopulmonary physiologic derangements that occur after this major operation.[22–25]

Additional factors

Besides pneumonectomy, some trials have attempted to identify other factors associated with perioperative changes in QoL. **Table 8** shows a summary of the findings of these investigations. Adjuvant chemotherapy[10,13] and age older than 70 years[11,14] were found to be associated with worse QoL, particularly with regard to physical domains. Open surgery (vs VATS)[15] and reduced DLCO[8] were also associated with poor physical recovery after surgery.

Pompili and colleagues[17] found that 3 months after lung resection, 28% of patients experienced a large decline in physical components and 15% of patients in mental components of QoL. Specific QoL domains were found to be associated with a perceived decline in physical status. In fact, better values for preoperative PF, for better bodily pain perception (less symptomatic), and for worse mental health were found to be associated with increased physical decline. The risk of perceived emotional decline was found to be greater in patients with lower predicted postoperative forced expiratory volume in 1 second (ppoFEV$_1$) and higher preoperative SF and mental health scores. The investigators used the SF36 survey for their analysis

Table 7
Standardized perioperative differences 12 months after pneumonectomy

Reference	Survey	No. of Patients	ES1	ES2	ES3	ES4	ES5	ES6
Balduyck et al[6]	EORTC	17	−0.49	−1.37	−0.67	−2.06	−0.47	−2.38
Schulte et al[14]	EORTC	16	0.24	−1.50	−0.21	n.r.	n.r.	−1.09
Kenny et al[16]	EORTC	25	0.12	−0.69	−0.50	−0.06	0.39	−0.57

An effect size of >0.8 (or <−0.8) is regarded as large, between 0.3 and 0.8 as medium, and <0.3 as small.

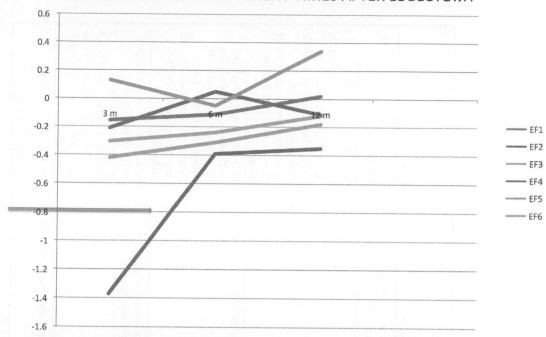

Fig. 1. Average values of effect sizes at different time points after pulmonary lobectomy. ES1, SF36 GH—general health perception or EORTC GHS—global health scale; ES2, SF36 physical functioning or EORTC physical functioning; ES3, SF36 social functioning or EORTC social functioning; ES4, SF36 MH—mental health or EORTC CF—cognitive functioning; ES5, SF36 RE—role limitation caused by emotional problems or EORTC EF—emotional functioning; ES6, SF36 RP—role limitation caused by physical problems or EORTC RF—role functioning. An effect size of greater than 0.8 (or <−0.8) is regarded as large, between 0.3 and 0.8 as medium, and less than 0.3 as small.

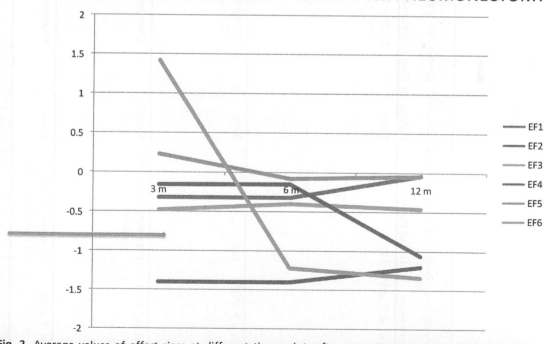

Fig. 2. Average values of effect sizes at different time points after pneumonectomy. ES1, SF36 GH—general health perception or EORTC GHS—global health scale; ES2, SF36 physical functioning or EORTC physical functioning; ES3, SF36 social functioning or EORTC social functioning; ES4, SF36 MH—mental health or EORTC CF—cognitive functioning; ES5, SF36 RE—role limitation caused by emotional problems or EORTC EF—emotional functioning; ES6, SF36 RP—role limitation caused by physical problems or EORTC RF—role functioning. An effect size of greater than 0.8 (or <−0.8) is regarded as large, between 0.3 and 0.8 as medium, and less than 0.3 as small.

Table 8
Summary of evidence related to factors associated with perioperative changes of QoL scales

Reference, Year	No. of Patients	Follow-Up Time	Outcome	Methods	Main Results
Pompili et al,[17] 2011	172	3 mo	Decline in SF36 PCS and MCS	Logistic regression and bootstrap analysis. Decline measured by effect size	Factors associated with a large decline in PCS: high preoperatively physical functioning, high bodily pain, and low mental health scores. Factors associated with a large decline in MCS: low ppoFEV1, high preoperative scores of social functioning and mental health
Handy et al,[8] 2002	103	6 mo	Changes in SF36 and QLI scales	Univariable group analysis	DLCO <45% was associated with worse postoperative SF36 RF and BP and with worse QLI overall QoL, health and functioning, and psychological or spiritual subscales
Handy et al,[9] 2010	192 OPEN vs 49 VATS patients	6 mo	Changes in SF36 scales	Retrospective unmatched comparison	Compared with open surgery, VATS determined a significantly lower negative impact on PF (−1.4 vs −11.6), RF (+12 vs −18.6), BP (+9.6 vs −4.4), GH (+4.4 vs −3.3)
Leo et al,[11] 2010	41 patients after pneumonectomy	6 mo	Changes in EORTC scales	Logistic regression analysis	Age >70 (OR 1.13) was associated with worse postoperative QoL

Study	N	Time	Measure	Analysis	Results
Sartipy[13] 2009	117	6 mo	Changes in SF36 scales	Logistic regression analysis	Adjuvant chemotherapy was associated with a decrease in ΔPCS%
Schulte et al,[15] 2009	131	Up to 24 mo	Changes in EORTC scales	Univariable group comparison elderly vs younger patients	Age >70 had worse values for PF, RF, and SF at 12–24 mo compared with younger patients
Kenny et al,[16] 2008	173	Up to 24 mo	Changes in EORTC scales	Group comparison (recurrence vs no recurrence) and linear regression analysis	Patients with recurrence had greater deterioration of overall QoL, PF, EF, pain, and fatigue compared with patients without recurrence at every time from 6 up to 24 mo postoperatively
Moller et al,[10] 2011	213	6 mo	Changes in SF36 scales	Logistic regression analysis	Extent of resection (OR 2.58) and adjuvant chemotherapy (OR 2.39) were associated with worse PCS (−10% from preoperative values). No factors associated with the decline in MCS

Abbreviation: OR, odds ratio.

and proposed the following regression equations to estimate the risk of a large decline in Physical Composite Scale and Mental Composite Scale.

Risk of physical decline: $\ln R/(1 + R)$: $-11.6 + 0.19 \times PF + 0.046 \times BP - 0.049 \times MH$

where PF = physical functioning, BP = bodily pain, MH = mental health scale scores.

Risk of emotional decline: $\ln R1/(1 + R1)$: $-8.06 - 0.03 \times ppoFEV_1 + 0.11 \times SF + 0.055 \times MH$

where SF = social functioning, MH = mental health scale scores.

SUMMARY

This article aims to evaluate the impact of pulmonary resection on residual QoL by means of a systematic quantitative review of the literature. Pulmonary lobectomy was found to have a transient influence on PF with subsequent partial recovery over time. No other scales were affected. By contrast, pneumonectomy had a large impact on physical and emotional domains. These scales did not show any recovery during follow-up, and many of them declined even more over time. In light of these findings, every effort should be made to avoid this type of surgery whenever technically and oncologically feasible.

ACKNOWLEDGMENTS

The authors would like to thank the conductors of the trials included in this article. In particular, they thank Bram Balduyck and Paul Van Schil and their coauthors; John R. Handy and his coauthors; Tobias Schulte and his coauthors; and Patricia M. Kenny and her coauthors. These investigators supplied invaluable unpublished data, without which this study could not have been completed.

REFERENCES

1. Lim E, Baldwin D, Beckles M, et al. Guidelines on the radical management of patients with lung cancer. Thorax 2010;65(Suppl 3):iii1–27.
2. Brunelli A, Charloux A, Bolliger CT, et al. ERS/ESTS clinical guidelines on fitness for radical therapy in lung cancer patients (surgery and chemo-radiotherapy). Eur Respir J 2009;34(1):17–41.
3. Brunelli A, Socci L, Refai M, et al. Quality of life before and after major lung resection for lung cancer: a prospective follow-up analysis. Ann Thorac Surg 2007;84(2):410–6.
4. Koller M, Kussman J, Lorenz W, et al. Symptom reporting in cancer patients: the role of negative affect and experienced social stigma. Cancer 1996;77(5):983–95.
5. Pompili C, Brunelli A, Xiumé F, et al. Prospective external convergence evaluation of two different quality-of-life instruments in lung resection patients. Eur J Cardiothorac Surg 2011;40(1):99–105.
6. Balduyck B, Hendriks J, Lauwers P, et al. Quality of life evolution after lung cancer surgery: a prospective study in 100 patients. Lung Cancer 2007;56:423–31.
7. Burfeind WR Jr, Tong BC, O'Branski E, et al. Quality of life outcomes are equivalent after lobectomy in the elderly. J Thorac Cardiovasc Surg 2008;136(3):597–604.
8. Handy JR, Asaph JW, Skokan L, et al. What happens to patients undergoing lung resection? Outcomes and quality of life before and after surgery. Chest 2002;122:21–30.
9. Handy JR, Asaph JW, Douville EC, et al. Does video-assisted thoracoscopic lobectomy for lung cancer provide improved functional outcomes compared with open lobectomy? Eur J Cardiothorac Surg 2010;37(2):451–5.
10. Moller A, Sartipy U. Predictors of postoperative quality of life after surgery for lung cancer. J Thorac Oncol 2012;7(2):406–11.
11. Leo F, Scanagatta P, Vannucci F, et al. Impaired quality of life after pneumonectomy: who is at risk? J Thorac Cardiovasc Surg 2010;139(1):49–52.
12. Pompili C, Brunelli A, Refai M, et al. Does chronic obstructive pulmonary disease affect postoperative quality of life in patients undergoing lobectomy for lung cancer? A case-matched study. Eur J Cardiothorac Surg 2010;37(3):525–30.
13. Sartipy U. Prospective population-based study comparing quality of life after pneumonectomy and lobectomy. Eur J Cardiothorac Surg 2009;36(6):1069–74.
14. Schulte T, Schniewind B, Dohrmann P, et al. The extent of lung parenchyma resection significantly impacts long-term quality of life in patients with non-small cell lung cancer. Chest 2009;135:322–9.
15. Schulte T, Schniewind B, Walter J, et al. Age-related impairment of quality of life after lung resection for non-small cell lung cancer. Lung Cancer 2010;68(1):115–20.
16. Kenny PM, King MT, Viney RC, et al. Quality of life and survival in the 2 years after surgery for non small-cell lung cancer. J Clin Oncol 2008;26(2):233–41.
17. Pompili C, Brunelli A, Xiumé F, et al. Predictors of postoperative decline in quality of life after major lung resections. Eur J Cardiothorac Surg 2011;39(5):732–7.
18. Salati M, Brunelli A, Xiumè F, et al. Quality of life in the elderly after major lung resection for lung cancer. Interact Cardiovasc Thorac Surg 2009;8(1):79–83.
19. Cohen J. Statistical power for the behavioral sciences. 2nd edition. Hillsdale (NJ): Lawrence Erlbaum Associates; 1988.

20. Valentine JC, Cooper H. Effect size substantive interpretation guidelines: issues in the interpretation of effect sizes. Washington, DC: What Works Clearinghouse; 2003.

21. Cykert S, Kissling G, Hansen CJ. Patient preferences regarding possible outcomes of lung resection: what outcomes should preoperative evaluations target? Chest 2000;117:1551–9.

22. Brunelli A, Xiumé F, Refai M, et al. Evaluation of expiratory volume, diffusion capacity, and exercise tolerance following major lung resection: a prospective follow-up analysis. Chest 2007;131(1):141–7.

23. Venuta F, Sciomer S, Andreetti C, et al. Long-term Doppler echocardiographic evaluation of the right heart after major lung resections. Eur J Cardiothorac Surg 2007;32(5):787–90.

24. Foroulis CN, Kotoulas CS, Kakouros S, et al. Study on the late effect of pneumonectomy on right heart pressures using Doppler echocardiography. Eur J Cardiothorac Surg 2004;26(3):508–14.

25. Alexiou C, Beggs D, Onyeaka P, et al. Pneumonectomy for stage I (T1N0 and T2N0) nonsmall cell lung cancer has potent, adverse impact on survival. Ann Thorac Surg 2003;76(4):1023–8.

Minimally Invasive Lung Surgery and Postoperative Quality of Life

John R. Handy Jr, MD, HonD

KEYWORDS

- Minimally invasive lung surgery • Quality of life • Lung cancer

KEY POINTS

- Patient priorities after medical intervention are, first and foremost, return to reasonable heath-related functional outcomes and quality of life (QOL). Undesired outcomes are permanent enfeeblement and, especially, cognitive impairment. Intervention will be declined if these poor outcomes are probable.
- Lung cancer patients are typically elderly, with a history of cigarette smoking; they have multiple comorbidities, tend to be less educated, and undergo large operations in hospitals to achieve cure. Any of these factors can predispose the patient to poor post-therapy functional status or cognitive dysfunction.
- Lung cancer surgery is associated with decreased health-related functional status and QOL for a variable length of time after surgery.
- Minimally invasive lung surgery mitigates or ameliorates the postoperative decline of health-related functional status and QOL.
- Little information addresses health-related functional outcomes or QOL after other types of commonly performed lung surgery such as decortication or pneumothorax.

In the United States in 2009 1,294,000 operations were performed on the respiratory system.[1] Therefore, quality of life (QOL) after lung surgery is clearly an important, but understudied, outcome.[2] To appreciate the potential impact of minimally invasive surgery (MIS) on the thoracic surgery (TS) patient's QOL, one must first understand the preferences and functional status of the patient at the onset of therapy as well as after treatment. Post-therapy QOL is being increasingly studied and proposed as a major end point in oncology trials and clinical evaluation.[2,3] Indeed, QOL deficits at the time of lung cancer diagnosis have been linked to survival.[4] So too in lung cancer surgery, QOL as determined by health-related functional status—both at baseline and subsequent postoperative

decline—correlated with survival.[5] The importance of the subject, finally, leads to proposed directions in research into QOL after TS. The existing literature pertains mainly to surgery for lung cancer and less so to other common thoracic diseases such as empyema, pneumothorax, or emphysema.

PATIENT PRIORITIES AFTER LUNG CANCER SURGERY

For decades, thoracic surgeons have focused on understanding, predicting, and managing operative mortality and complications as, admittedly, important end points to both the patient and surgeon. Operative morbidity and mortality have been the focus of innumerable medical articles

Conflict of interest: None.
Providence Thoracic Oncology Program, Providence Cancer Center, North Tower, 4805 Northeast Glisan Street, Portland, OR, USA
E-mail address: john.handy@providence.org

Thorac Surg Clin 22 (2012) 487–495
http://dx.doi.org/10.1016/j.thorsurg.2012.07.010
1547-4127/12/$ – see front matter

and the initial driver in the development of professional databases.[6] Other outcomes have evolved, often driven by payors, such as readmission to intensive care, reoperation, hospital length of stay (LOS), discharge disposition, and hospital readmission. Are these the outcomes that most concern the patient?

The short answer is no. Cykert and colleagues,[7] in a landmark study using outpatients awaiting appointments, examined patient preferences regarding possible outcomes of lung resection by evaluating postoperative complications (pneumonia, atelectasis, myocardial infarction), prolonged debility (progressively longer ventilator dependency, oxygen dependence) or permanent enfeeblement or incapacitation (limited walking ability, need of assistance with activities of daily living (ADLs), permanent ventilator dependency, and permanent nursing home placement). They used health utility scores in which 1.0 equals perfect health and 0 equals death (**Table 1**). They found patients ranked perioperative complications 0.49 to 0.81, while prolonged debility or permanent enfeeblement or incapacitation ranked 0.16 to 0.33 (least desirable). Progressive lung cancer also ranked 0.17. In short, the patient desires to be cured of the lung cancer and to return to as near normal activity as possible. Patients do not desire perioperative complications, but would not decline surgery due to them. The authors point out the irony of the surgical literature's focus on predicting complications during the perioperative period, which is almost always a transient state, as opposed to the patient perspective of avoiding permanent debility.

These findings are borne out in the larger (but still surprisingly small) literature concerning patient preferences and serious illness. Fried and colleagues[8] reported on 226 patients having cancer, chronic obstructive lung disease, or congestive heart failure (each contributing about one-third to the study population), evaluating burden of treatment (high vs low) and return to current health, severe functional impairment, or severe cognitive impairment. Note the end point of return to current health versus normal or preillness health in this sick population. Surgery was defined as 1 of the high burden scenarios. In the case of low burden and return to current health, 98.7% desired treatment. If treatment was high burden but return to current health, 88.8% desired treatment. However, for low burden and severe functional impairment or severe cognitive impairment, only 25.6% and 11.2% of patients, respectively, wanted treatment. There

Table 1
Patients' perception of possible outcomes of lung surgery as represented by utility scores

Outcomes	Utility Score[a] (95% Confidence Interval)
Pneumonia requiring 2 wk of hospitalization	0.81 (0.74–0.88)
Atelectasis requiring bronchoscopic therapy	0.80 (0.72–0.88)
Ventilator dependence for 3 d	0.76 (0.68–0.84)
Ventilator dependence for 7 d	0.74 (0.66–0.82)
Ventilator dependence for 15 d	0.66 (0.57–0.75)
Ventilator dependence for 30 d	0.59 (0.49–0.69)
Permanent ventilator dependence with estimated survival of 6 mo	0.10 (0.04–0.16)
Acute myocardial infarction	0.49 (0.40–0.59)
Can walk only 2 city blocks without stopping	0.48 (0.40–0.56)
Current activity level reduced by half	0.44 (0.37–0.51)
Oxygen dependence	0.33 (0.26–0.40)
1 mo of nursing home placement followed by a 1-block walking limitation (because of dyspnea)	0.30 (0.23–0.37)
Need assistance with ADLs	0.19 (0.13–0.25)
Limited to bed-to-chair existence	0.17 (0.11–0.23)
Progressive lung cancer	0.17 (0.10–0.24)
Permanent nursing home placement	0.16 (0.10–0.22)

[a] Utility scores range from 0 representing death to 1 representing perfect health.
Data from Cykert S, Kissling G, Hansen CJ. Patient preferences regarding possible outcomes of lung resection: what outcomes should preoperative evaluations target? Chest 2000;117:1553.

was no significant difference across diagnostic categories. Interestingly, the percentage desiring to be treated decreased as the probability of adverse outcome increased, but the reductions were greater for disability than death. When the adverse outcome was death, the number of participants substantially decreased only when the likelihood was 90% or more. For functional or cognitive disability, the substantial decrease began at 50% likelihood. These same investigators found at 2-year follow-up, either more time or a declining health status further decreased willingness to undergo highly burdensome treatment or risk severe disability to avoid death.[9]

The enhanced undesirability of cognitive versus functional impairment mentioned has precedent. A wonderfully entitled article, "Fates worse than death," by Ditto and colleagues,[10] studied 2 populations (college students and elderly) and found both groups viewed health states characterized by cognitive dysfunction more negatively than either physical or sensory dysfunction. Health state alternatives were evaluated through the lens of valued life activities (VLA). In both groups' VLAs, the ability to engage in social relations was rated highest. They summarized that cognitive dysfunction was most disruptive of VLAs, producing very low QOL ratings and low interest in life-sustaining therapies.

Summarizing, patients desired to be cured of lung cancer and wish to avoid permanent functional, but above all, cognitive impairment. Death is preferable to severe permanent cognitive impairment. In other words, the long-term patient goals of lung cancer resection are improved length of life with an acceptable quality.

FUNCTIONAL STATUS OF LUNG CANCER SURGERY PATIENTS

Lung cancer patients have worse performance status than other cancer patients. The relative risk of poor performance status in localized lung cancer (ie, potentially resectable) is 3 times that of a localized breast cancer patient, while advanced lung cancer is 5 times higher.[11] This study compared 500 lung cancer patients to 2885 other cancer patients, including breast, colon, head and neck, and lymphoma and prostate cancer patients. Lung cancer patients were at the highest risk for poor performance status compared with patients who had the other common cancers. Importantly, providers tended to underestimate poor performance status.

As lung cancer occurs in cigarette smokers and is dose related, older people with associated smoking-related diseases get the disease.[12–14]

Further, lung cancer surgery, being physiologically impactful, is performed in hospitals. How do older patients with multiple diseases fare in hospitals or with large surgery?

Sager and colleagues[15] conducted a multicenter prospective cohort study of 1279 community-living patients older than 70 years hospitalized for acute nonsurgical illness. ADLs were determined at admission, discharge, and 3 months after discharge. Additionally, Mini-Mental State Examination was performed at admission to determine cognition. Discharge diagnoses included circulatory system (26%), respiratory system (20%), digestive system (15%), cancer (6%), and other (33%). At discharge, 59% of patients reported no change; 10% improved, and 31% declined in ADLs compared with preadmission. At 3 months, 11% of patients died, and 40% reported new ADL disabilities. The 3-month outcomes were the result of loss of function during hospitalization, failure to recover after discharge, and development of new postdischarge disabilities. Greatest risk for adverse functional outcomes was found in older, preadmission ADL disabilities or lower mental status on admission, and also with rehospitalization.

Hansen and colleagues[16] conducted a study 1 month after discharge of patients older than 65 years who were independent in their ADLs before hospitalization and were dependent at discharge (home nursing). Admission was for acute nonsurgical, nonpsychiatric medical illness, including pneumonia, congestive heart failure, ischemic heart disease, gastrointestinal disease, and chronic obstructive pulmonary disease. They found the likelihood of recovery of independence was high (76%) if

> No in-door assist device was required prior to hospitalization
>
> Patients had a good Mini-Mental State Examination result and timed "up and go" of less than 20 seconds

If any 1 of these elements was poor, the patient was unlikely to recover independence within 1 month (poor cognition: 87% not recovered, indoor assist device: 85%, timed "up and go" >40 seconds: 73%) **Fig 1**.

Major noncardiac surgery without complications has been associated with postoperative cognitive decline. Using neurocognitive testing, Duke investigators reported 44.8% of 29 patients undergoing noncardiac surgery demonstrated cognitive decline 6 to 12 weeks postoperatively.[17] The majority of the 29 patients underwent TS (lobectomy –11 patients, wedge resection–6 patients, pneumonectomy–2 patients, decortication–1 patient, and chest wall

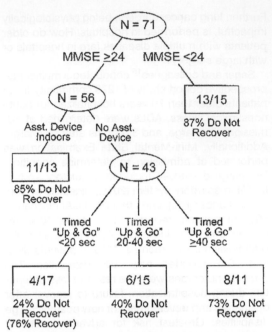

Fig. 1. Algorithm showing results of a study conducted 1 month after discharge of patients older than 65 years who were independent in their ADLs before hospitalization and were dependent at discharge (home nursing). *Abbreviation:* MMSE, Mini-Mental State Examination. *(From Hansen K, Mahoney J, Palta M. Risk factors for lack of recovery of ADL independence after hospital discharge. J Am Geriatr Soc 1999;47:363; with permission.)*

resection–1 patient). Forty-five percent of lobectomy patients and 66% of wedge resection patients experienced cognitive decline. Multivariate analysis showed age (odds ratio 2 for each decade) and years of education (1.6% improvement for each year of education) to be predictors of cognitive decline.

Price and colleagues[18] studied a cohort of 337 surgery patients older than 60 years and 60 controls at baseline, at discharge, and 3 months afterward using cognitive and ADL instruments. Surgery breakdown was as follows: 50 MIS, 167 intra-abdominal/thoracic, and 138 orthopedic. Fifty-six percent experienced cognitive decline at discharge, with equal distribution in type and severity. At 3 months, 75% of patients had no decline; 13.6% had only memory decline. Executive function decline was reported in 8.4% of patients, and 2.9% had both memory and executive function decline. Memory decline was not associated with functional decline, but executive function decline and combined memory and executive function decline were. Of those with decline, 46.8% of cases were mild; 32.5% were moderate, and 20.8% were severe. Patients with combined memory and executive impairment were significantly less educated

than patients with either memory or executive impairment alone.

Lung cancer survivors, presumably most from surgery, although no information was given in the article, have more problems than other cancer survivors.[19] A cross-sectional study of disease-free lung, and colon and prostate cancer survivors showed no difference in global, physical, psychosocial, medical interaction, marital, or sexual QOL variables between short- versus long-term lung cancer survivors at an average of 3.4 years after diagnosis. However, lung cancer survivors had frequent and severe problems with ADLs, working, pain, psychological distress, cognitive function, sexual function, marital relations, medical interactions, and communication and interaction with partners compared with colon and prostate cancer survivors. Predictors of QOL for lung cancer survivors included only performance status and work status. These authors concluded cancer survivors do not return to a normal state of health. With this as a background, smoking or former-smoker lung cancer survivors are at high risk for new second primary lung cancers and potential candidates for additional surgery.[20]

Approximately 20% of Americans smoke cigarettes regularly.[21] Among cancer survivors, 15% are current smokers.[22] Active smoking contributes to poor QOL whether young and healthy or after lung cancer surgery. In healthy young smokers (university students), there were lower mean QOL scores overall compared with nonsmokers, but these were especially significant in physical functioning, general health, energy, social functioning, and mental health.[23] In a European study, current smoking at the time of lung cancer surgery (50% of study population), showed no return to baseline values 12 months postoperatively in physical functioning, social functioning, and persistent dyspnea. Additionally, patients experienced increased thoracic pain.[24] For nonsmokers (13% of study population), QOL returned to baseline at 3 months postoperatively in all parameters.

In short, lung cancer surgery patients, by virtue of their age, habits, and comorbidities, are at risk for functional decline from their habits, disease, or hospitalization. Also, lung cancer patients are at risk for cognitive impairment from lung surgery, perhaps even increased risk due to the characteristically lower educational level of smokers.[25]

Is this not this exactly what patients seeking cure are trying to avoid?

QOL AND MIS LUNG CANCER SURGERY

Lung cancer surgery patients start off disadvantaged. QOL for preoperative lung cancer patients is inferior to that of the healthy population.[26] Preoperative lung cancer patients have significantly worse physical functioning, emotional, mental, and energy subscales compared with matched normals.

At 6 months after surgery using open surgical approaches for pulmonary resection, physical functioning, pain, and mental health were worse than preoperatively.[26] Variations on these deficits are in multiple publications using various validated instruments to evaluate postlung resection QOL. After major lung resection, worsening has been reported for physical and mental components at 3 months,[27] physical functioning and dyspnea at 1 year,[28] and physical functioning, pain, dyspnea, and fatigue at 2 years.[29,30] Age and gender have no effect on postoperative QOL,[28,30-32] but larger extent of pulmonary resection (pneumonectomy) has a disproportionly persistent worsening of physical component.[29,33] Also, poor preoperative diffusion capacity,[26] preoperative dyspnea, adjuvant chemotherapy, age,[34,35] and disease recurrence (36% of stage 1 and 2 patients)[36] have been cited as predictive of poorer postlung resection QOL.

Technical improvements have been called for to positively affect postlung resection QOL.[26] MIS could be such an improvement.

Video-assisted thoracic surgery (VATS) lobectomy has many technical forms and has been slow in universal adoption.[37] Meanwhile, VATS lobectomy has evolved into a totally endoscopic approach.[38] Recent reports concerning 5-year oncologic equivalency of thoracoscopic lobectomy[39] and a propensity-matched analysis of the Society of Thoracic Surgeons (STS) general thoracic database demonstrating lower incidence of complications of thoracoscopic lobectomy compared with open lobectomy pose a compelling argument for MIS lobectomy to be the standard of care for lung cancer surgery.[40] What about functional status and QOL, since these are the patients' priorities?

Studies using nonpatient-reported outcomes imply functional recovery after VATS lobectomy is superior. A report of lobectomy in octogenarians showed not only that the VATS patients had a shorter LOS (5 vs 6 days, $P = .001$), but only 5% of VATS were discharged to rehabilitation versus 22.5% of thoracotomy patients ($P = .015$).[41] VATS lobectomy patients have been reported as better recipients of adjuvant chemotherapy compared with thoracotomy.[42] There were fewer delays (18% vs 58%) and fewer reduced doses (26% vs 49%). Additionally, 61% of VATS patients received 75% of planned regimen without delay or reduced dose compared with 40% of thoracotomy patients.

Others have interpreted similar information to infer superior functional outcomes and QOL from thoracoscopic lobectomy.[43]

The few patient-reported outcomes published confirm the superiority of thoracoscopic versus open lobectomy regarding functional status and QOL. None of the studies was randomized, which is characteristic of postoperative QOL literature. In 2007, Aoki and colleagues compared 16 thoracotomy to 17 VATS lobectomy patients by mailing the 36-Item Short Form Health Survey (SF36), a validated long-standing instrument measuring general health-related functional status and commonly used in many of the prior listed reports,[26] 3, 12, and 36 months postoperatively.[44] They found quicker recovery in the VATS patients. In 2002, Li and colleagues[45] reported on 27 VATS major lung resection patients versus 24 thoracotomy patients out to 33 to 39 months using the European Organization for Research and Treatment of Cancer (EORTC) instruments. They found VATS patients tended to score higher on QOL and functioning scales, report fewer symptoms, and take less pain medicine, but the differences were not significant.

In 2007, Balduyck and colleagues[46] reported 100 patients undergoing "major pulmonary surgery for malignant disease." Overall, of the 61 lobectomies, only 1 was performed with VATS, and of the 22 wedge resections, 7 were performed with VATS. Patients were administered EORTC instruments at 1, 3, 6, 12 months after surgery. They found lobectomy and wedge resections fared similarly with decrease QOL and increase pain at 1 month and more dyspnea for lobectomy patients. By 3 months, all parameters had returned to baseline, except pain for lobectomy. Pneumonectomy patients (17, no VATS) remained significantly below baseline at 12 months in physical functioning, pain, shoulder function, and dyspnea. VATS patients were significantly better than thoracotomy patients in physical functioning, pain, and QOL at all points measured.

In a prospective observational study reported in 2010, Handy and colleagues[47] compared VATS lobectomy patients (49) to open patients (192) preoperatively and 6 months postoperatively using multiple clinical parameters and the SF-36. Only lobectomy was analyzed, thus ensuring a uniform loss of pulmonary parenchyma in the study population. The VATS group had better preoperative pulmonary function testing, more adenocarcinoma, and lower stage. The VATS patients versus open patients did not differ regarding operating time, postoperative complications, hospital mortality, or 6 month mortality. VATS patients had less blood loss, transfusion, and intraoperative fluid administration and shorter LOS (5.2 vs 6.6 days, P = .03). At 6 months after surgery, VATS patients were either at baseline or better in all 8 SF36 categories (physical functioning, role functioning–physical, role functioning–emotional, social functioning, bodily pain, mental health, energy, and general health), while open patients were significantly worse than baseline in physical functioning, role functioning–physical, and social functioning **Fig. 2**. VATS patients had fewer hospital readmissions, less use of pain medicine, and better preservation of preoperative performance status.

This small body of literature appears to verify that MIS TS provides what patients desire, equal probability of cure, superior postoperative functional recovery, and return to presurgery functional status.

EMPYEMA, PNEUMOTHORAX, EMPHYSEMA

Much less literature addresses these common thoracic diseases, which are often treated with TS. Treatment for empyema has eluded being translated into a simple algorithim.[48] Early surgical therapy for advanced cases (greater than American Thoracic Society stage 2A, fibrinopurulent with loculations and no pleural peel) leads to superior results,[49] is cost-effective,[50] and commonly performed with substantial morbidity and mortality.[51] Few reports compare open surgery versus VATS, with most simply demonstrating feasibility with VATS.[52–54] A large nonrandomized report comparing VATS with open decortication, in not exactly comparable patients, shows less operative time,

postoperative air leak, atelectasis, reintubation, ventilator dependency, transfusion, sepsis, LOS, and 30-day mortality in favor of VATS.[55] No studies address functional status or QOL. An Italian study of 123 thoracotomies versus 185 VATS decortications did note earlier return to work with VATS (25 ± 5.2 days vs 34.1 ± 9.9 days; P<.0001),[56] which is a very plausible QOL surrogate.

Pneumothorax is a common thoracic malady with a defined role for surgical treatment. Open treatment has the lowest recurrence rate (1% vs 5%), but VATS is better tolerated and generally recommended.[57,58] VATS has reduced LOS, fewer analgesic requirements and, perhaps, less postoperative pulmonary dysfunction.[59] A Venezuelan report on 53 thoracotomy patients versus 47 VATS patients treatment of spontaneous primary pneumothorax, found at 3 years 97% of VATS considered themselves "completely recovered" versus 79% in open. Chronic or intermittent pain requiring narcotics greater than once a month occurred in 90% open versus 13% VATS. Finally, 13% of thoracotomy patients required "clinical pain management" while no VATS patients had this requirement.[60] Only 1 paper addressed QOL after surgery for pneumothorax. Baldyck and colleagues[61] followed 20 consecutive patients undergoing wedge resection and apical pleurectomy (9 patients with VATS and 11 with anterolateral thoracotomy) with serial testing using EORTC instruments over 1 year. All patients' cough & dyspnea improved postoperatively. The QOL indicators were not different except at 1 month when VATS had improved physical, role, cognitive functioning, and dyspnea.

Emphysema surgery, or lung volume reduction surgery (LVRS) is seldom performed despite having level 1 evidence supporting improvement in survival, exercise capacity, and QOL in the appropriate patient population.[62,63] The National Emphysema Treatment Trial (NETT), which generated the evidence most convincingly, allowed both VATS and median sternotomy approaches and provided long-term follow up.[64] Complication rates were low for both, and mortality was equal.[65] VATS has shorter LOS, less cost of operation and hospitalization, better independent living by 30 days after surgery (80.9% vs 70.5%), and less cost in the 6 months after surgery. Functional outcomes were not different at 12 and 24 months. This information has been interpreted as defining VATS as the preferred approach due to earlier recovery and lower cost.[66] VATS has become the primary approach in the few centers that have remained focused on LVRS.[67] The NETT gathered data on health-related QOL, general QOL, and dyspnea, but analysis comparing VATS to open has never been published.[64]

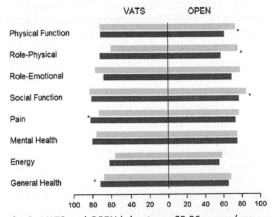

Fig. 2. VATS and OPEN lobectomy SF-36 scores (gray = preoperative, black = postoperative, 0 = worst; 100 = best, * P = 0.05). (From Handy JR, Asaph JW, Douville EC, et al. Does video-assisted thoracoscopic lobectomy for lung cancer provide improved functional outcomes compared with open lobectomy? Eur J Cardiothorac Surg 2010;37:453; with permission.)

FUTURE RESEARCH DIRECTIONS IN FUNCTIONAL STATUS AND QOL AFTER TS

QOL after surgery (or any treatment) is the primary focus of the patient seeking cure or symptomatic improvement. QOL assessment should be comprehensive of all TS interventions, not just lobectomy. Large populations must be studied. Given the patient primacy of functional recovery, postoperative TS prediction formulae should be developed from preoperative variables and validated. Cognitive function and return to work should also be assessed, as these are important to the patient. TS QOL research needs to be more longitudinal, inclusive of multiple early, midterm, and long-term time points to be able to discern the trajectory of recovery. If recovery is systematically incomplete, causes can be hypothesized and studied. Remediation should be then proposed and studied for efficacy. Patient satisfaction after TS has not been approached at all. Computer or Internet direct patient entry could diminish cost, improve access, lessen travel, and lead to more complete data when using questionnaires and QOL instruments, especially over long timeframes.

Postoperative QOL research is a rich area of potential investigation, which can be contributed to by busy clinicians and does not require large monetary investment. Additionally, unlike the less common outcomes of postoperative mortality or morbidity, every surviving patient has functional, cognitive, and QOL outcomes; thus much smaller study populations are required to achieve statistical significance, confirming or refuting hypotheses. Given the importance of the subject and the paucity of existing information, anyone with interest and focus can become an expert in the field.

REFERENCES

1. Prevention Fastats homepage. Available at: http://www.cdc.gov/nchs/fastats/insurg.htm. Accessed June 9, 2012.
2. Gralla RJ. Coming of age for monitoring quality of life and patient-reported outcomes. J Thorac Oncol 2012;7:8–9.
3. Brunelli A, Charloux A, Bollinger CT, et al. The European Respiratory Society & European Society of Thoracic Surgeons clinical guidelines for evaluating fitness for radical treatment (surgery & chemotherapy) in patients with lung cancer. Eur J Cardiothorac Surg 2009;36:181–4.
4. Sloan JA, Zhao X, Novotny PJ, et al. Relationship between deficits in overall quality of life and non-small cell lung cancer survival. J Clin Oncol 2012; 30:1498–504.
5. Moeller A, Sartipy U. Association between changes in quality of life and survival after lung cancer surgery. J Thorac Oncol 2012;7:183–7.
6. Caceres M, Braud RL, Garrett HE. A short history of the Society of Thoracic Surgeons National Cardiac Database: perception of a practicing surgeon. Ann Thorac Surg 2010;89:332–9.
7. Cykert S, Kissling G, Hansen CJ. Patient preferences regarding possible outcomes of lung resection: what outcomes should preoperative evaluations target? Chest 2000;117:1551–9.
8. Fried TR, Bradley EH, Towle VR, et al. Understanding the treatment preferences of seriously ill patients. N Engl J Med 2002;346:1061–6.
9. Fried TR, Van Ness PH, Byers AL, et al. Changes in preferences for life-sustaining treatment among older persons with advanced illness. J Gen Intern Med 2007;22:495–501.
10. Ditto PH, Druley JA, Smucker WD, et al. Fates worse than death: the role of valued life activities in health-state evaluations. Health Psychol 1996; 15:332–43.
11. Lilenbaum RC, Cashy J, Hensing TA, et al. Prevalence of poor performance status in lung cancer patients: implications for research. J Thorac Oncol 2008;3:125–9.
12. Raviv S, Hawkins KA, DeCamp MM, et al. Lung cancer in chronic obstructive pulmonary disease. Am J Respir Crit Care Med 2011;183:1138–46.
13. Tammemagi CM, Neslund-Dudas C, Smioff M, et al. In lung cancer patients, age, race-ethnicity, gender and smoking predict adverse comorbidity, which in turn predicts treatment & survival. J Clin Epidemol 2004;57:597–609.
14. De Torres JP, Marin JM, Casanova C, et al. Lung cancer in patients with chronic obstructive pulmonary disease: incidence and predicting factors. Am J Respir Crit Care Med 2011;184:913–9.
15. Sager MA, Franke T, Inouye SK, et al. Functional outcomes of acute medical illness and hospitalization in older persons. Arch Intern Med 1996;156:645–52.
16. Hansen K, Mahoney J, Palta M. Risk factors for lack of recovery of ADL independence after hospital discharge. J Am Geriatr Soc 1999;47:360–5.
17. Grichnik KP, Ijsselmuiden AJ, D'Amico TA, et al. Cognitive decline after major noncardiac operations: a preliminary prospective study. Ann Thorac Surg 1999;68:1786–91.
18. Price CC, Garvan CW, Monk TG. Type & severity of cognitive decline in older adults after noncardiac surgery. Anesthesiology 2008;108:8–187.
19. Shag CA, Ganz PA, Wing DS, et al. Quality of life in adult survivors of lung, colon and prostate cancer. Qual Life Res 1994;3:127–41.
20. Asaph JW, Keppel JF, Handy JR, et al. Surgery for second lung cancers. Chest 2000;118:1621–5.

21. Poll G. Available at: http://www.gallup.com/poll/109048/us-smoking-rate-still-coming-down.aspx?version=print. Accessed June 11, 2012.

22. Underwood JM, Townsend JS, Stewart L, et al. Surveillance of demographic characteristics & health behaviors among adult cancer survivors—Behavioral Risk Factor Surveillance System, United States, 2009. MMWR Surveill Summ 2012;61:1–23.

23. Martinez JA, Mota GA, Vianna ES, et al. Impaired quality of life of healthy young smokers. Chest 2004;125:425–8.

24. Balduyck B, Nia PS, Cogen A, et al. The effect of smoking cessation on quality of life after lung cancer surgery. Eur J Cardiothorac Surg 2011;40:1432–8.

25. Garrett BE, Dube SR, Trosclair A, et al. Cigarette smoking—United States, 1965–2008. MMWR Surveill Summ 2011;60:109–13.

26. Handy JR, Asaph JW, Skokan L, et al. What happens to patients undergoing lung cancer surgery? Outcomes and quality of life before and after surgery. Chest 2002;122:21–30.

27. Pompili C, Brunelli A, Siume F, et al. Predictors of postoperative decline in quality of life after major lung resections. Eur J Cardiothorac Surg 2011;39:732–7.

28. Balduyck B, Hendriks J, Lauwers P, et al. Quality of life evolution after lung cancer surgery in septuagenarians: a prospective study. Eur J Cardiothorac Surg 2009;35:1070–5.

29. Schulte T, Schniewind B, Dohrmann P, et al. The extent of lung parenchyma resection significantly impacts long-term quality of life in patients with non-small cell lung cancer. Chest 2009;135:322–9.

30. Ferguson MK, Parma CM, Celaura AD, et al. Quality of life and mood in older patients after major lung resection. Ann Thorac Surg 2009;87:1007–13.

31. Sartipy U. Influence of gender on quality of life after lung surgery. Eur J Cardiothorac Surg 2010;37:802–6.

32. Moeller A, Sartipy U. Changes in quality of life after lung surgery in old and young patients: are they similar? World J Surg 2010;34:684–91.

33. Sartipy U. Prospective population-based study comparing quality of life after pneumonectomy and lobectomy. Eur J Cardiothorac Surg 2009;36:1069–74.

34. Paull DE, Thomas ML, Meade GE, et al. Determinants of quality of life in patients following pulmonary resection for lung cancer. Am J Surg 2006;192:565–71.

35. Moeller A, Sartipy U. Predictors of postoperative quality of life after surgery for lung cancer. J Thorac Oncol 2012;7:406–11.

36. Kenny PM, King MT, Viney RC, et al. Quality of life and survival in the 2 years after surgery for non-small cell lung cancer. J Clin Oncol 2008;26:233–41.

37. Rocco G, Internull E, Cassivi SD, et al. The variability of practice in minimally invasive thoracic surgery for pulmonary resections. Thorac Surg Clin 2008;18:235–47.

38. Hartwig MG, D'Amico TA. Thoracoscopic lobectomy: the gold standard for early stage lung cancer? Ann Thorac Surg 2010;89:2098–101.

39. Yamamoto K, Ohsumi A, Kojima F, et al. Long-term survival after video-assisted thoracic surgery lobectomy for primary lung cancer. Ann Thorac Surg 2010;89:353–9.

40. Paul S, Altorki NK, Sheng S, et al. Thoracoscopic lobectomy is associated with lower morbidity than open lobectomy: a propensity-matched analysis from the STS database. J Thorac Cardiovasc Surg 2010;139:366–78.

41. Port JL, Mira FM, Lee PC, et al. Lobectomy in octogenarians with non-small cell lung cancer: ramification of increasing life expectancy and the benefits of minimally invasive surgery. Ann Thorac Surg 2011;92:1951–7.

42. Petersen RP, Pham DK, Burfeind W, et al. Thoracoscopic lobectomy facilitates the delivery of chemotherapy after resection for lung cancer. Ann Thorac Surg 2007;83:1245–50.

43. Demmy TL, Nwogu C. Is video-assisted thoracic surgery lobectomy better? Quality of life considerations. Ann Thorac Surg 2008;85:S719–28.

44. Aoki T, Tsuchida M, Hashimoto T, et al. Quality of life after lung cancer surgery: video-assisted thoracic surgery vs thoracotomy. Heart Lung Circ 2007;16:285–9.

45. Li WW, Lee TW, Lam SS, et al. Quality of life following lung cancer resection: video-assisted thoracic surgery vs thoracotomy. Chest 2002;122:584–9.

46. Balduyck B, Hendriks J, Van Schil P. Quality of life evolution after lung cancer surgery: a prospective study of 100 patients. Lung Cancer 2007;56:423–31.

47. Handy JR, Asaph JW, Douville EC, et al. Does video-assisted thoracoscopic lobectomy for lung cancer provide improved functional outcomes compared with open lobectomy? Eur J Cardiothorac Surg 2010;37:451–5.

48. Molnar TF. Current surgical treatment of thoracic empyema in adults. Eur J Cardiothorac Surg 2007;32:422–30.

49. Wozniak CJ, Paull DE, Moezzi JE, et al. Choice of first intervention is related to outcomes in the management of empyema. Ann Thorac Surg 2009;87:1525–31.

50. Thourani VH, Brady KM, Mansour KA, et al. Evaluation of treatment modalities for thoracic empyema: a cost-effectiveness analysis. Ann Thorac Surg 1998;66:1121–7.

51. Farjah F, Symons RG, Krishnadasan B, et al. Management of pleural space infections: a population-based analysis. J Thorac Cardiovasc Surg 2007;133:346–51.

52. Mackinlay TA, Lyon GA, Chimondeguy DJ, et al. VATS debridement vs thoracotomy in the treatment

of loculated post-pneumonia empyema. Ann Thorac Surg 1996;61:1626–30.

53. Roberts JR. Minimally invasive surgery in the treatment of empyema: intraoperative decision making. Ann Thorac Surg 2003;76:225–30.

54. Solaini L, Prusciano F, Bagioni P. Video-assisted thoracic surgery in the treatment of pleural empyema. Surg Endosc 2007;21:280–4.

55. Tong BC, Hann J, Toloza EM, et al. Outcomes of video-assisted thoracoscopic decortication. Ann Thorac Surg 2010;89:220–5.

56. Cardilla G, Carleao F, Carbone L, et al. Chronic post-pneumonic pleural empyema: comparative merits of thoracoscopic vs open decortication. Eur J Cardiothorac Surg 2009;36(5):914–8.

57. Baumann MH, Strange C, Heffner JE, et al. Management of spontaneous pneumothorax: an American College of Chest Physicians Delphi consensus statement. Chest 2001;119:590–602.

58. MacDuff A, Arnold A, Harvey J. Management of spontaneous pneumothorax: British Thoracic Society pleural disease guideline 2010. Thorax 2010;65:ii18–31.

59. Vohra HA, Adamson L, Weeden DF. Does video-assisted thoracoscopic pleurectomy result in better outcomes than open pleurectomy for primary spontaneous pneumothorax? Interact Cardiovasc Thorac Surg 2008;7:673–7.

60. Olavarrieta JR, Coronel P. Expectations & patient satisfaction relate to the use of thoracotomy and video-assisted thoracoscopic surgery for treating recurrence of spontaneous primary pneumothorax. J Bras Pneumol 2009;35:122–8.

61. Baldyck B, Hendriks J, Lauwers P, et al. Quality of life evolution after surgery for primary or secondary spontaneous pneumothorax: a prospective study comparing different surgical techniques. Interact Cardiovasc Thorac Surg 2008;7:45–9.

62. Sanchez PG, Kucharczuk JC, Su S, et al. National Emphysema Treatment Trial redux: accentuating the positive. J Thorac Cardiovasc Surg 2010;140:564–72.

63. Criner GJ, Cordova F, Sternberg AL, et al. The NETT part II: lessons learned about lung volume reduction surgery. Am J Respir Crit Care Med 2011;184:881–93.

64. Fishman A, Martinz F, Naunheim K, et al. A randomized trail comparing lung volume reduction surgery with medical therapy for severe emphysema. N Engl J Med 2003;348:2059–73.

65. McKenna RJ, Benditt JO, DeCamp M, et al. Safety and efficacy of median sternotomy vs video-assisted thoracic surgery for lung volume reduction surgery. J Thorac Cardiovasc Surg 2004;127:1350–60.

66. Huang W, Wand WR, Deng B, et al. Several clinical interests regarding lung volume reduction surgery for sever emphysema: meta-analysis and systematic review of randomized controlled trials. J Cardiothorac Surg 2011;6:148–56.

67. Ginsburg ME, Thomashow BM, Yip CK, et al. Lung volume reduction surgery using the NETT selection criteria. Ann Thorac Surg 2011;91:1556–61.

Quality of Life in the High-Risk Candidate for Lung Resection

Sabha Ganai, MD, PhD[a], Mark K. Ferguson, MD[b],*

KEYWORDS

- Quality of life • Thoracic • Lung resection • High-risk • Decision analysis

KEY POINTS

- Compared with patients with other cancer types, lung cancer patients have significant impairments at baseline, from the ability to conduct activities of daily living to global quality-of-life (QOL) measures.
- Analysis of functional outcomes after lung resection demonstrates significant impairments in QOL parameters after pneumonectomy, but otherwise no striking differences in QOL based on the few other high-risk features studied.
- The elderly do not have a significant detriment in QOL with surgery, despite baseline impairments in physical functioning.
- The data support the value of tailoring an individualized approach that is compatible with the preferences and goals of the patient, regardless of their risk of surgical complications, as long as the patient comprehends the nature and likelihood of those risks.

We should always let our judgments and recommendations be guided by the fact that we operate on patients, not on diseases.
—*Stanley O. Hoerr, MD[1]*

Despite the prospect of long-term survival in select patients amenable to pulmonary resection, the likelihood of perioperative morbidity and mortality may be considered prohibitive in those with significant cardiopulmonary risk.[2,3] While surgery is only offered to 16% to 21% of patients presenting with lung cancer,[4,5] it is a management decision that is typically based upon a composite of favorable characteristics determined by tumor and patient. Patient and physician perception of risk, including that attributed to age and perceived longevity, can further influence choices among therapeutic strategies.

Shared decision making entails a model in which clinicians and patients achieve agreement about medically appropriate treatment options after discussion of the risks, benefits, and the level of uncertainty of each option, all in context with the patient's preferences and values.[6] Critical examination of the values and preferences of patients with lung cancer suggest that the optimal choice of therapy may not be purely based on standard outcome measures such as expected 5-year survival, but should consider the morbidity, adverse effects, and convenience of the treatment, as well as personal attitudes toward risk taking and values attributed toward possible perioperative death and death from the disease itself.[7] Treatment-related and cancer-related symptoms including fatigue, pain, dyspnea, cough, hemoptysis, and anorexia play an important role in the quality of life (QOL) of

The authors have nothing to disclose.
a Department of Surgery, The University of Chicago Medical Center, 5841 South Maryland Avenue, MC 6040, Chicago, IL 60637, USA; b Department of Surgery and Cancer Research Center, The University of Chicago Medical Center, 5841 South Maryland Avenue, MC 5040, Chicago, IL 60637, USA
* Corresponding author. The University of Chicago Medical Center, 5841 South Maryland Avenue, MC 5040, Chicago, IL 60637.
E-mail address: mferguso@surgery.bsd.uchicago.edu

lung cancer patients.[8] Recent evidence that patient-reported QOL at the time of diagnosis is a prognosticator of survival reaffirms the importance in addressing the physical, psychological, and social elements of lung cancer care and their implications on health outcomes.[9,10] This article provides perspective on how known and estimated measures of QOL influence treatment decisions in patients who are high-risk candidates for lung resection.

DEFINING THE HIGH-RISK CANDIDATE

The assessment of perioperative risk remains a challenge even for expert surgeons, with risk estimates in clinical practice established by a composite of subjective and objective criteria.[11] Optimal patient selection for therapeutic options requires an understanding of the risk–benefit ratio of each option and an appreciation of the possibility of complications that may be attributed to known pretreatment clinical variables considered as risk factors. Analysis of 18,800 patients reported by participants of the Society of Thoracic Surgeons (STS) General Thoracic Surgery Database from 2002 to 2008 revealed numerous variables predictive of major morbidity (7.9% incidence) and mortality (2.2% incidence) after resection for lung cancer, as summarized in **Table 1**.[12] Diffusing capacity of the lung for carbon monoxide (DLCO) was not included in their multivariate model due to missing data in 40% of patients. However, diminished DLCO has an established association with morbidity and mortality after pulmonary resection,[13,14] as well as recently defined implications on long-term survival after resection for cancer.[15,16]

While several risk models for determining the likelihood of perioperative mortality have been developed from large databases,[17–19] they provide limited data on prediction of the relative risk of complications. For these composite measures to be clinically meaningful as decision tools, they should ideally allow stratification of patients into groups at high risk of complications and prohibitive risk of in-hospital mortality. Further investigation in the methodology of risk assessment is expected, but currently leads the authors to resort to expert opinion and smaller datasets in determining thresholds for decision making.

A joint multidisciplinary task force of the European Respiratory Society and the European Society of Thoracic Surgeons recently presented guidelines on assessment for fitness for both surgery and chemoradiotherapy in patients with lung cancer.[20] Guidelines included the performance of lung cancer surgery by qualified thoracic surgeons in adequate-volume centers under the management of multidisciplinary teams. Recommendations were also

Table 1
Significant predictors of perioperative morbidity and mortality after lung cancer resection[a]

Predictors of Major Morbidity (8%)	Predictors of Mortality (2%)
Performance status	Performance Status
ASA score (4 or 5)	ASA score
Pneumonectomy or bilobectomy (vs wedge resection)	Dialysis use
Lobectomy, sleeve lobectomy, or segmentectomy (vs wedge resection)	Pneumonectomy or bilobectomy (vs wedge resection)
Induction chemoradiotherapy	Creatinine >2
Dialysis use	Induction chemoradiotherapy
Creatinine >2	Pathologic stage IV
Steroid use	Steroid use
Thoracotomy vs VATS	Age
Congestive heart failure	Urgent or emergent vs elective case
Recent cigarette use	Male gender
Age	BMI (inversely proportional)
BMI (inversely proportional)	FEV$_1$ (inversely proportional)
Coronary artery disease	
FEV$_1$ (inversely proportional)	

Abbreviations: ASA, American Society of Anesthesiologists; BMI, body mass index; DLCO, diffusing capacity of the lung for carbon monoxide; FEV$_1$, forced expiratory volume in the first second of expiration; VATS, video-assisted thoracoscopic surgery.

[a] Note that DLCO and clinical staging were excluded from analysis due to missing data. Data with significance of $P<.05$ are included and were ranked according to their odds ratio.

Data from Kozower BD, Sheng S, O'Brien SM, et al. STS database risk models: predictors of mortality and major morbidity for lung cancer resection. Ann Thorac Surg 2010;90:878.

provided for preoperative cardiac assessment and perioperative risk reduction, as well as routine pulmonary function testing with estimation of predicted postoperative forced expiratory volume in the first second of expiration (FEV$_1$) and DLCO. Either value less than 30% of predicted is considered a high-risk threshold in the assessment of pulmonary reserve before surgery.

In 2010, the British Thoracic Society and the Society for Cardiothoracic Surgery in Great Britain and Ireland updated their guidelines, recommending a tripartite risk assessment using:

1. The 2007 American College of Cardiology/American Heart Association guidelines for perioperative cardiovascular evaluation[21] to assess for risk of postoperative cardiac events,
2. A global risk score such as Thoracoscore[18] to assess for risk of perioperative death,
3. Dynamic pulmonary function testing with measurement of DLCO to assess for risk of postoperative dyspnea.[22]

Moderate to high risk of dyspnea was stratified according to a predicted postoperative FEV_1 and/or DLCO less than 40%, similar to clinical practice guidelines published by the American College of Chest Physicians.[23] However, surgical resection was still recommended as an option for patients with moderate to high risk of postoperative dyspnea as long as these patients are properly informed of their risks of dyspnea, long-term oxygen requirement, and associated complications.

While risk assessment adds great value by allowing for informed choices based on a desire to avoid possible morbidity and mortality, decision making is not always based on objective criteria in the clinical arena. Objective measures such as those obtained from cardiac evaluation and pulmonary function testing are helpful for determining that a patient may be inoperable, but even those otherwise considered operative candidates have other forms of risk that may be simply determined by the gestalt obtained from an expert clinician. These composite measures, however, may also be subject to considerable bias based on numerous misconceptions of risk, including chronologic age, which may be influenced to different degrees at an individual level by the impact of physiologic changes, associated comorbidities, and functional status.[24,25]

Significant underrepresentation of elderly patients is recognized in cancer clinical trials, with the greatest barrier being physician perception about age and tolerability of treatments.[26] Age also appears to inappropriately influence recommendations for therapy in clinical settings outside of clinical trials.[27] Frailty is a concept that explores the global decrease in physiologic reserve with age and has become the subject of recent investigation in geriatric populations, with particular interest in defining methodology to quantify and modify its impact on surgical outcome.[25,28] Frailty and disability metrics have been shown to accurately predict in-hospital morbidity and mortality in high-risk elderly patients undergoing cardiac surgery.[29,30] The criteria required for optimal clinical decision making and determination of risk in thoracic patients, especially among the elderly, remain worthy topics of further investigation.

DETERMINANTS OF QOL AFTER LUNG RESECTION

Health-related QOL is a multidimensional concept encompassing social, emotional, cognitive, physical, and functional well-being.[8] While preoperative risk evaluation allows for assessment of patient safety before undergoing surgery, QOL assessments allow for evaluation of these other elements in the context of the patient's global functioning. While QOL changes may be cancer-related, such as the emotional and psychosocial distress imparted by a diagnosis of cancer and diminished projected lifespan, postoperative decline in QOL may also be influenced by treatment-related events, such as the requirement of additional therapies or procedures (eg, opening wound, bronchoscopy, stenting, tube thoracostomy, or reoperation), prolonged or new symptoms (eg, pain, dyspnea, neuropathy, or hoarseness), and disturbances in social life (eg, delay of return to employment, performance status decline, impact on family life, or loss of independence).[8,31]

Numerous validated QOL instruments are available, including general QOL scales like the 36-Item Short Form Health Survey (SF-36) (**Box 1**)[32] and cancer-specific QOL scales such as the European Organization for Research and Treatment of Cancer (EORTC) Quality of Life Questionnaire (QLQ-C30 (**Box 2**).[33] Both instruments have well-established reliability and validity, with the

---

Box 1
Elements of the SF-36

Physical health dimensions
- Physical functioning
- Role limitations due to physical problems
- Bodily pain
- General health perceptions

Mental health dimensions
- Mental functioning
- Role limitations due to emotional problems
- Social functioning
- Vitality

Data from Ware JE, Sherbourne CD. The MOS 36-item short-form health survey (SF-36). Med Care 1992;30: 473–83.

Box 2
Elements of the EORTC QLQ-C30 health survey

Functioning scales

- Physical
- Role
- Cognitive
- Emotional
- Social
- Global quality of life

Symptom scales and other items

- Fatigue
- Nausea and vomiting
- Pain
- Dyspnea
- Sleep disturbance
- Appetite loss
- Constipation
- Diarrhea
- Financial impact

Data from Aaronson NK, Ahmedzai S, Bergman B, et al. The European Organization for Research and Treatment of Cancer QLQ-C30: a quality of life instrument for use in international clinical trials of oncology. J Natl Cancer Inst 1993;85:365–77.

SF-36 having applicability in a wide range and severity of conditions,[32,34,35] while the EORTC QLQ-C30 is often paired with a lung-specific questionnaire, allowing assessment of symptoms specifically geared toward patients with lung cancer.[33,36]

Clinical trials examining traditional outcomes such as overall survival after chemotherapy in advanced lung cancer have more frequently been using QOL endpoints, with hopes that QOL measures may influence selection of treatments with similar survival.[37] However, QOL is a dynamic concept, with changes over time that may be influenced by treatment effects, alterations in the disease situation, as well as psychological phenomena including adaption, coping, expectancy, and optimism.[38,39] Part of the value of studying QOL may be gained by the performance of repeated assessments in a longitudinal fashion and gaining understanding of the short-term and long-term consequences of these treatment decisions. QOL as a measure is even more complex than previously understood, and may even be influenced by genetic predisposition, as distinct single nucleotide polymorphisms have been shown to be associated with pain, fatigue, and

overall QOL in heterogeneous populations of lung cancer patients.[40]

Using the EORTC QLQ instruments, Zieren and colleagues[41] demonstrated that patients undergoing lung resection had dysfunction in physical functioning and role functioning (performance of job and household tasks) that returned to baseline by 9 to 12 months after surgery. Of importance, patients undergoing lobectomy had better physical functioning and less dyspnea than patients undergoing pneumonectomy, although no significant differences in global QOL were seen between the 2 types of lung resection. Recent prospective analysis of lobectomy and pneumonectomy patients using the SF-36 confirmed that pneumonectomy patients experience significant declines in physical functioning and vitality scores at 6 months postoperatively.[42] In addition, using the EORTC QLQ instrument, Schulte and colleagues[43] have shown that significant decreases in physical and social functioning occur within 3 to 6 months of pneumonectomy, with more pain, dyspnea, and coughing. Similarly, Balduyck and colleagues found that elderly patients undergoing pneumonectomy had worse physical functioning, role functioning, social functioning, and general pain scores.[44]

Using the SF-36 and quality of life index (QLI) instruments, Handy and colleagues[45] analyzed the influence of lung cancer surgery on QOL, examining several possible risk factors for perioperative morbidity. Preoperatively, patients already had a decrease in most QOL measures when compared with age-matched healthy controls. At 6 months after lung resection, physical functioning, social functioning, mental health, and bodily pain subscales were significantly worsened compared with preoperative values. Of note, preoperative DLCO below 45% was a significant predictor of both poor preoperative and postoperative QOL, with significant deficits in health and functioning, psychological, and overall QOL subscales. Postoperative QOL was not influenced by preoperative FEV_1, ability to perform a 6-minute walk, use of induction or adjuvant therapy, extent of resection, or postoperative complications.

Pompili and colleagues[46] recently performed an analysis of QOL before and after lobectomy for lung cancer in patients with chronic obstructive pulmonary disease (COPD). Patients with COPD had significantly lower FEV_1, DLCO, comorbidity index, and performance status than the non-COPD cohort. Using propensity score case-matched pairs, comparisons were made demonstrating no significant differences in preoperative and postoperative QOL scales using the SF-36 instrument. Despite poor preoperative respiratory function and an increased risk of postoperative complications, patients with COPD were found to have similar QOL measures compared with the general population.

Brunelli and colleagues[47] prospectively evaluated QOL before and after lung resection for non-small cell lung cancer (NSCLC) using the SF-36 taken along with pulmonary function and stair climbing tests at 1 and 3 months postoperatively. Physical composite scores were decreased at 1 month, but returned to baseline at 3 months, while no changes were noted in mental composite scores. Examining subgroups of high-risk patients, including male gender, age older than 70 years, COPD, DLCO less than 70%, postoperative predicted FEV_1 or DLCO less than 40%, or coronary artery disease, no significant differences were seen in physical and mental composite scores. Patients undergoing pneumonectomy were found to experience significant declines at 3 months in physical composite scores when compared with patients who underwent lobectomy. Poor correlation was seen between physical and mental composite scores and the FEV_1, DLCO, and height reached on stair climbing measured during each evaluation period. Discrepancies may exist between patient perceptions of QOL and these objective measures, and patient-reported QOL may be argued to be of more value for intervention than those objective criteria. Overall, it remains unclear if high-risk patients have any significant detriment in QOL after lobectomy, suggesting that surgical management may still be offered despite risk of perioperative complications and mortality in the context of the patient's preferences and understanding of these risks and benefits.

THE INFLUENCE OF AGE ON QOL

Examination of the National Cancer Database revealed that treatment choices for lung cancer in the United States in 2001 were predicted by stage and age; patients who were 70 years or older were less likely to be treated surgically than younger patients, regardless of stage, and comorbid conditions primarily influenced treatment choices for patients with more advanced disease.[5] In that year, 51% of patients diagnosed with NSCLC in the United States were over 70 years of age. Seventy-two percent of patients had at least 1 comorbid condition, with 27% of patients having COPD. Among stage I patients (25%), 72% were treated surgically, with elderly patients significantly less likely to receive surgery than younger patients. An analysis of the Surveillance, Epidemiology, and End Results (SEER) cancer registry similarly showed that patients with lung cancer who were younger than 70 years received cancer-directed surgery more than 70% of the time, in comparison to only 40% of patients over 80 years of age.[48]

Reeve and colleagues[49] recently analyzed linked data from the SEER cancer registry and the Medicare Health Outcomes Survey (MHOS), examining health-related QOL measures in cancer patients over 65 years at a population-based level. The linked SEER-MHOS dataset allowed for paired propensity score matching between these cancer patients and cancer-free control subjects. Of 9 examined cancer types in patients on Medicare, those with NSCLC had the greatest decline in physical health. Furthermore, lung cancer patients showed the greatest decline in ability to perform activities of daily living in comparison to control subjects, especially bathing, dressing, eating, getting in and out of chairs, and using a toilet. Only lung cancer patients demonstrated statistically significant changes in mental health and bodily pain in comparison to controls. Lung cancer patients also had significant decreases in social function, vitality (ie, fatigue), and general health perceptions, and overall these patients had the greatest decline in all measures of health-related QOL.

Patients in the SEER database with lung cancer were reported as having cancer-directed surgery for curative intent in 67% of cases. Surgery was not recommended (physician belief that surgery was not the best treatment option) in 17% of cases, contraindicated (medical contraindication) in 6% of cases, refused (patient belief that surgery was not the best treatment option) in 3% cases, and unknown in 7% of cases.[48] The reporting of not recommended was significantly predicted by an age over 75 years, as well as by tumor size and black or Hispanic race. The rationale behind physicians not recommending curative surgery and whether this is appropriate is unclear, but further exploration of the reasons physicians do not offer surgery based on age is warranted, especially if the elderly receive similar benefit when controlled for comorbidity and functional status.[50] Physician refusal may be based on skepticism and bias rather than data.

Salati and colleagues[51] reported QOL measures in patients older and younger than 70 years of age after major resection for lung cancer. Preoperatively, elderly patients had decreased ability to climb stairs, as well as differences in American Society of Anesthesiologists (ASA) score and Eastern Cooperative Oncology Group (ECOG) performance status. Using the SF-36, elderly patients were significantly lower in physical functioning but had higher mental health scores in comparison to the younger cohort preoperatively.

At 3 months after the operation, there were no significant differences between younger and older patients across all QOL metrics. Moreover, their data suggest that QOL in elderly returns to preoperative values within 3 months of an operation. Within the elderly group, assessing for high-risk features including DLCO less than 70%, COPD, predicted postoperative FEV$_1$ or DLCO less than 40%, coronary artery disease, or pneumonectomy revealed no significant differences in QOL measures.

Schulte and colleagues[52] examined QOL in elderly patients undergoing lobectomy for NSCLC using the EORTC QLQ lung cancer-specific instruments. Examining physical functioning, they found that younger patients had greater declines in QOL scores at discharge and 3 months, while older patients were only impacted after a 2-year interval. Younger patients suffered more from pain at all time points. Dyspnea scores were better in older patients up to 6 months, but differences evened out by 2 years. All patients demonstrated an improvement in coughing by 6 months, with no significant differences seen between age groups. Regarding social functioning scales, at discharge, younger patients were worse off, but quickly improved, with decreases in social functioning in older patients at 2 years. Likewise, role functioning scales were worse in young patients at discharge, and decreased in older patients at 6-, 12-, and 24-month time points. Overall global health scales showed that young patients fare worse in QOL at discharge, while older patients approximate their preoperative QOL by 12 months. While young patients demonstrated actual improvements in QOL after lobectomy at 12 and 24 months compared with their preoperative state, elderly patients simply returned to their baseline.

Burfeind and colleagues[53] used the EORTC QLQ instrument in a prospective, longitudinal fashion to assess their patients undergoing lobectomy and found no significant difference between older (>70 years) and younger cohorts. Both groups experienced significant reductions in physical functioning, role functioning, social functioning, and global QOL at 3 months, but by 6 months, QOL domains had returned to baseline. Moreover, emotional functioning was less impaired at all time points in older patients.

Ferguson and colleagues[54] reported QOL outcomes of elderly patients after recovery from major lung resection using the EORTC QLQ lung cancer-specific instruments and the Depression Anxiety Stress Scale (DASS-21) questionnaire. Older patients (≥70 years) had higher rates of prior myocardial infarction and COPD at baseline, and had a significantly higher incidence of postoperative complications. However, at more than 6 months after surgery, there were no significant differences in QOL between age cohorts, although the elderly trended toward having poorer physical function, more fatigue, greater dyspnea, and less depression than younger patients. On multivariate analysis, covariates for QOL, symptom, and mood scores included pulmonary complications, which predicted worse physical function scores, and low percent predicted postoperative FEV$_1$, which corresponded with worse physical function, role function, pain, fatigue, and dyspnea scores. Meaningful evaluations of the role of DLCO could not be made due to the majority of patients analyzed having no impairments in this measure.

Examination of QOL in long-term lung cancer survivors showed significant decline with time in measures of pain, fatigue, and dyspnea when compared between short-term (<3 year) and long-term (>5 year) assessments.[55] Factors significantly associated with poor QOL at short-term follow-up included male gender, squamous cell carcinoma, and poor fatigue and pain scores. Older age, cancer progression or recurrence, and poor scores in fatigue, dyspnea, and pain were independent predictors of poor long-term QOL.

Overall, elderly patients appear to experience similar physical, emotional, and social consequences from lung resection when compared with the general population.[50] While they may have greater baseline physical dysfunction, they also appear to have greater emotional resiliency than their younger counterparts, and may have different subjective responses to pain. Most studies reviewed showed a return of QOL scores toward a preoperative baseline from 3 to 9 months after surgery. While young patients tend to have more acute changes in QOL at discharge, older patients appeared to have more long-term impairments at a year or longer. Whether these are directly related to lung resection or a consequence of evolving physiologic and functional changes remains uncertain.

TREATMENT OPTIONS AND ALTERNATIVES FOR HIGH-RISK PATIENTS

While lobectomy with systematic lymph node evaluation has been established as the standard of care for management of early stage NSCLC, high-risk patients are often offered several less-morbid treatment options, including sublobar resection, external beam radiation therapy, stereotactic beam radiation therapy (SBRT), and percutaneous ablative therapies.[56,57] Each of these therapies has tradeoffs that typically include accepting an increased risk of locoregional recurrence and cancer-related death for lower rates of perioperative death and complications. In the context of placing value on functional outcomes and QOL over survival, these therapies may serve as viable alternatives in high-risk patients based on patient preferences.

In 1995, The Lung Cancer Study Group trial concluded that limited resection has higher rates of death and locoregional recurrence in comparison with lobectomy, and does not necessarily confer improved perioperative morbidity, mortality, or postoperative function.[58] However, the role of sublobar resection on postoperative QOL has only been studied in a limited fashion. Balduyck and colleagues[59] showed no significant changes in global QOL in patients who underwent wedge resection, with only minor decreases at 1 month in physical functioning, role functioning, and social functioning. While lobectomy patients had an increase in dyspnea in the first month postoperatively, patients undergoing wedge resection had no change in dyspnea or coughing scores, and had similar changes in pain scores and greater shoulder dysfunction at 1 month after surgery. Recent analysis of 2090 patients in the SEER database with stage I NSCLC less than or equal to 1cm in size found that limited resections were performed in a third of patients, and were more likely to be performed in older patients.[60] Regression analysis could not identify differences in overall survival between lobectomy and sublobar resection in the entire cohort and age-stratified subgroups, suggesting that sublobar resection may be a viable alternative in moderate- to high-risk patients with small tumors. This question is now being prospectively addressed as the subject of the Cancer and Leukemia Group B (CALGB) 140503 trial in patients at all risk levels.

Combining wedge resection with adjuvant mesh brachytherapy may be an alternate strategy to decrease local recurrence through an additional intervention during the same operation.[61] The American College of Surgeons Oncology Group (ACOSOG) Z4032 trial recently reported baseline and 3-month functional outcomes in 148 high-risk patients with stage 1 NSCLC randomized to sublobar resection with and without brachytherapy, finding no clinically meaningful differences in DLCO, FEV_1, or dyspnea scores.[62] Follow-up of their primary endpoint, local recurrence, is still required to establish any conclusions, but from a QOL perspective, little advantage or detriment is noted from adjuvant brachytherapy at short-term assessment.

Thoracoscopic lobectomy has been shown to result in similar postoperative QOL when compared with open lobectomy when assessed by the EORTC QLQ instruments.[63] Balduyck and

colleagues[59] demonstrated that thoracoscopic approaches were actually more favorable in terms of their evolution of physical functioning, role functioning, and global QOL at 6 months, with less pain and shoulder dysfunction compared with the experience of patients undergoing thoracotomy. Propensity-matched analysis of the STS database demonstrated a reduction in complications such as arrhythmias and reintubation, with lower chest tube duration and shorter length of stay with video-assisted thoracoscopic lobectomy.[64] Thoracoscopy has been considered the method of choice of resection specifically for elderly patients based on improved postoperative outcomes.[65] The role of minimally invasive techniques to specifically manage higher-risk patients appear promising from both a morbidity and QOL perspective, and they will certainly define themselves as practice patterns evolve to accommodate their greater use.

While external beam radiation, SBRT, and ablative therapies have traditionally been limited to inoperable patients, their use has been extended to operable patients at high risk of complications from surgery.[66] In inoperable patients with stage I NSCLC undergoing 3-dimensional conformal radiotherapy (3D-CRT) or SBRT, QOL has been assessed using the EORTC instruments.[67] No significant changes have been noted over time in global QOL or physical functioning after SBRT, although dyspnea increased slightly. Significantly worse declines were noted in physical functioning after 3D-CRT in comparison to SBRT. Moreover, overall survival in inoperable patients undergoing 3D-CRT was 48% at 2 years, which was significantly less than 72% at 2 years for SBRT. Overall, SBRT appears to have greater advantages over 3D-CRT across QOL and survival outcome measures.

Onishi and colleagues[68] examined 87 patients with operable stage I NSCLC who refused surgery and underwent high-dose hypofractionated SBRT with a biologically effective dose over 100 Gy. Favorable 5-year local control rates of 92% and 73% and 5-year overall survival of 72% and 62% were seen in patients with stage IA and IB disease, respectively. A recent study of clinical stage I NSCLC patients treated with surgery or SBRT revealed no significant differences in overall survival, disease-specific survival, or local control among propensity-matched subgroups, despite overall survival differences at 3 years of 68% and 32%.[69] SBRT was performed in significantly older patients with more comorbidities and a lower predicted FEV_1 and DLCO, with morbidity including grade 1–2 pneumonitis in 52% of patients, grade 3 pneumonitis in 1% of patients, and other minor complications (eg, rib fracture or pleural effusions) in 14% of patients. However, the matched subgroup of high-risk surgical patients had an operative mortality of 7% and morbidity of 44%, including 21% with arrhythmias and 27% with pneumonia and respiratory failure. SBRT may prove to be a promising alternative to lung resection in select tumors, especially in similar high-risk patients. Survival and QOL outcomes in high-risk patients randomized to SBRT versus sublobar resection (with or without brachytherapy) are current subjects of the ACOSOG Z4099 trial.

Radiofrequency ablation (RFA) and microwave ablation are emerging modalities in the local treatment of lung cancer in patients with metastatic disease, as well as high-risk, early stage patients with small, peripheral tumors.[70] The RAPTURE study, a prospective, multicenter trial evaluating the efficacy of RFA for pulmonary lesions, assessed QOL and functional outcomes of patients with metastatic disease and primary NSCLC who were otherwise considered inoperable and not amenable to radiotherapy or chemotherapy.[71] They found no significant worsening in pulmonary function tests over a year of follow-up, with similar QOL outcomes at baseline and 12 months. Further assessment of QOL outcomes comparing the different alternative treatments is warranted before any conclusions can be made beyond standard outcomes like survival benefit.

THE ROLE OF DECISION ANALYSIS FOR HIGH-RISK PATIENTS

Decision analysis methodology remains a useful tool for the study of replicated medical conditions of uncertainty in which probabilities and tradeoffs are explicitly addressed.[72] Decision models, however, must be structured appropriately, providing all relevant therapeutic options and their outcomes with assigned probabilities for each health state as derived from relevant literature.[73] In situations where randomized clinical trials cannot be easily performed, decision analysis can be helpful to replicate numerous states of reality. Values or utilities are incorporated to allow parameters for decision making, and they can be tested across a range of uncertainty in the data. While useful, this may still be subject to bias based on the available studies reported describing the various health states. The perspective of the utility of those health states should also be considered, whether from the point of view of the patient or the health system (ie, cost-effectiveness).[74,75]

Cykert and colleagues[74] reported patient-rated health utility scores for various postoperative outcomes after lung resection, ranging from short-

and long-term ventilator dependence, oxygen dependence, nursing home placement, and changes in activity level. Older patients attributed less interest in temporary ventilator dependence than younger patients, and patients with poor self-rated health valued pneumonia, atelectasis, and ventilator dependence with lower utility compared with patients with good health. Conversely, those with good health scored the possibility of lung cancer progression much lower than patients who already considered themselves with poor health. It is possible that patients who are at high risk for perioperative morbidity will have similar attitudes toward complications that may guide their treatment decisions.

To determine the optimal use of alternative strategies for stage I NSCLC, a Markov model was used to simulate a 65-year old man with medically inoperable peripheral stage I NSCLC, providing the options of 3D-CRT, SBRT, and RFA.[76] Predicted 3-year overall survival rates were 31%, 44%, and 29%, respectively. From a cost-effectiveness perspective, SBRT was considered the most acceptable nonsurgical treatment modality, followed by RFA if unavailable. Markov modeling of cost-effectiveness of surgical intervention versus SBRT for high-risk patients with stage I NSCLC has suggested that SBRT may initially be a more cost-effective alternative to surgery in patients at high risk of complications, although because of the longer expected overall survival, surgical intervention may ultimately be the better decision.[77]

Another Markov model examined medically operable stage I NSCLC, comparing SBRT to lobectomy in groups with minor and major comorbidities using utilities based on patient perspectives.[78] Simulation of a 65-year old man with minor comorbidities predicted a 5-year overall survival of 67% for surgery versus 64% for SBRT. Modeling a 65-year old man with major comorbidities and heavy smoking predicted a 5-year overall survival of 57% for surgery versus 54% for SBRT. Overall analysis across gender and risk groups demonstrated a benefit of surgery over SBRT ranging from 2% to 3%. When assessing quality-adjusted life years, results were similar between lobectomy and SBRT, with differences ranging from 0.07 to 0.09 across all patient cohorts. Further population-based studies examining both cost and utility may assist in determining the best option for high-risk patients, but both SBRT and surgical approaches appear at least similar from both the patient and payor perspectives.

Uncertainty ultimately requires inferences of the situation with a determination of its value as a positive or negative, an opportunity or a danger.[38]

Patients tend to express risk aversion toward surgery, especially with a prospect of changes in functional status, physical disability, and loss of independence.[79] Risk-averse subjects often turn down gambles with positive expected value based on their prior beliefs in the payoffs of one strategy in comparison to the other.[80] Risk-averse patients who may favor a nonoperative decision pathway are influenced by their understanding of prognosis, diagnostic uncertainty, and perceptions of alternative therapies, requiring precision by clinicians in communicating data and potential outcomes. Decision tools may assist with elucidating a patient's preferences and guiding his or her choices.

BARRIERS TO ADDRESSING QOL AND PATIENT PREFERENCES

While QOL is an important construct in the management of lung cancer, assessment of QOL and functional outcomes is primarily done in the arena of clinical trials and in the context of academic study, not in community clinical practice.[8] Questionnaires are often considered time consuming and bothersome by patients, and they are prone to statistical problems related to missing data.[37] QOL measurements may also be biased toward a patient population that does not experience significant treatment-related complications or mortality based on the nature of follow-up. QOL data may be limited in patients exceeding thresholds for risk factors who could be considered inoperable by objective criteria, as they are naturally excluded from postoperative assessments when surgery is refused or denied. In addition, most QOL measurements are not compared with similar patients who do not undergo surgery or an alternate therapy, so the true impact of the therapy on QOL is unknown.

Furthermore, bias of clinicians in only offering certain treatments within their scope of practice may exist and limit provision of therapies in concert with a patient's preference, especially when management is not discussed in a multidisciplinary setting. Choices may be subject to framing bias, where a decision may be guided differently based on presentation of the likelihood of survival rather than a likelihood of death.[81] Therapy may also be simply not offered based on misconception of risk. In the scope of advanced lung cancer, there is a lower likelihood of receiving chemotherapy associated with age despite similar survival benefits in the elderly.[82] Older age remains a significant predictor of not being offered entry into a clinical trial when controlled for comorbidity and functional status.

Elderly patients who do participate in cancer clinical trials choose to do so based on a preference to obtain the best treatment available, an improvement in their health, and a possible cure for their cancer.[26] Both younger and older patients who refuse participation do so based on an interest in choosing their own treatment.[26,83] Such findings only stress the importance to consider patient preferences of the young and old. It is likely that in the context of lung resection, similar biases may be in practice as in the delivery of chemotherapy, requiring thoughtful and critical evaluation by clinicians into the rationale behind the treatment options they provide and choose to offer.

SUMMARY

No consensus exists for the optimal management of operable lung cancer in high-risk patients. Lung cancer patients have significant impairments at baseline, from ability to conduct activities of daily living to global QOL measures when compared with patients with other cancer types.[49] Analysis of functional outcomes after lung resection demonstrate significant impairments in QOL parameters after pneumonectomy, but otherwise no striking differences in QOL based on the few other high-risk features studied. Examination of the role of age suggests that the elderly do not have a significant detriment in QOL with surgery, despite baseline impairments in physical functioning. In fact, the data are supportive of the value of tailoring an individualized approach that is compatible with the preferences and goals of the patient, regardless of his or her risk of surgical complications, as long as the patient comprehends the nature and likelihood of those risks. Critical analysis of the methodology of risk assessment is still warranted, and as studies on functional outcomes and QOL are rather limited, future discourse may provide greater insight on how one can better counsel patients to make informed choices.

REFERENCES

1. Hoerr SO. Hoerr's law. Am J Surg 1962;103(4):411.
2. Brunelli A. Risk assessment for pulmonary resection. Semin Thorac Cardiovasc Surg 2010;22:2–13.
3. Fernandes EO, Teixeira C, Silva LC. Thoracic surgery: Risk factors for postoperative complications of lung resection. Rev Assoc Med Bras 2011;57:292–8.
4. Strand TE, Bartnes K, Rostad H. National trends in lung cancer surgery. Eur J Cardiothorac Surg 2012;42(2):355–8.
5. Little AG, Gay EG, Gaspar LE, et al. National survey of non-small cell lung cancer in the United States: epidemiology, pathology and patterns of care. Lung Cancer 2007;57:253–60.

6. Politi MC, Studts JL, Hayslip JW. Shared decision making in oncology practice: what do oncologists need to know? Oncologist 2012;17:91–100.

7. McNeil BJ, Weichselbaum R, Pauker SG. Fallacy of the five-year survival in lung cancer. N Engl J Med 1978;299:1397–401.

8. Pearman T. Psychosocial factors in lung cancer: quality of life, economic impact, and survivorship implications. J Psychosoc Oncol 2008;26:69–80.

9. Quinten C, Coens C, Mauer M, et al. Baseline quality of life as a prognostic indicator of survival: a meta-analysis of individual patient data from EORTC clinical trials. Lancet Oncol 2009;10:865–71.

10. Sloan JA, Zhao X, Novotny PJ, et al. Relationship between deficits in overall quality of life and non-small-cell lung cancer survival. J Clin Oncol 2012; 30:1498–504.

11. Ferguson MK, Stromberg JD, Celauro AD. Estimating lung resection risk: a pilot study of trainee and practicing surgeons. Ann Thorac Surg 2010; 89:1037–43.

12. Kozower BD, Sheng S, O'Brien SM, et al. STS database risk models: predictors of mortality and major morbidity for lung cancer resection. Ann Thorac Surg 2010;90:875–83.

13. Ferguson MK, Vigneswaran WT. Diffusing capacity predicts morbidity after lung resection in patients without obstructive lung disease. Ann Thorac Surg 2008;85:1158–64.

14. Ferguson MK, Gaissert HA, Grab JD, et al. Pulmonary complications after lung resection in the absence of chronic obstructive pulmonary disease: the predictive role of diffusing capacity. J Thorac Cardiovasc Surg 2009;138:1297–302.

15. Liptay MJ, Basy S, Hoaglin MC, et al. Diffusion lung capacity for carbon monoxide (DLCO) is an independent prognostic factor for long-term survival after curative lung resection for cancer. J Surg Oncol 2009;100:703–7.

16. Ferguson MK, Dignam JJ, Siddique J, et al. Diffusing capacity predicts long-term survival after lung resection for cancer. Eur J Cardiothorac Surg 2012;41:e81–6.

17. Berrisford R, Brunelli A, Rocco G, et al. The European Thoracic Surgery Database project: modeling the risk of in-hospital death following lung resection. Eur J Cardiothorac Surg 2005;28:306–11.

18. Falcoz PE, Conti M, Brouchet L, et al. The Thoracic Surgery Scoring System (Thoracoscore): risk model for in-hospital death in 15,183 patients requiring thoracic surgery. J Thorac Cardiovasc Surg 2007; 133:325–33.

19. Bernard A, Rivera C, Pages PB, et al. Risk model of in-hospital mortality after pulmonary resection for cancer: a national database of the French Society of Thoracic and Cardiovascular Surgery (Epithor). J Thorac Cardiovasc Surg 2011;141:449–58.

20. Brunelli A, Charloux A, Bollinger CT, et al. ERS/ESTS clinical guidelines on fitness for radical therapy in lung cancer patients (surgery and chemo-radiotherapy). Eur Respir J 2009;34:17–41.

21. Fleisher LA, Beckman JA, Brown KA, et al. ACC/AHA 2007 guidelines on perioperative cardiovascular evaluation and care for noncardiac surgery: a report of the American College of Cardiology/American Heart Association Task Force on Practice Guidelines. Circulation 2007;116:e418–99.

22. Lim E, Baldwin D, Beckles M, et al. Guidelines on the radical management of patients with lung cancer. Thorax 2010;65:iii1–27.

23. Colice GL, Shafazand S, Griffin JP, et al. Physiologic evaluation of the patient with lung cancer being considered for resectional surgery: ACCP evidenced-based clinical practice guidelines (2nd edition). Chest 2007;132:161S–77S.

24. Holmes HM. Quality of life and ethical concerns in the elderly thoracic surgery patient. Thorac Surg Clin 2009;19:401–7.

25. Fried LP, Tangen CM, Walston J, et al. Frailty in older adults: evidence for a phenotype. J Gerontol A Biol Sci Med Sci 2001;56:M146–56.

26. Townsley CA, Selby R, Siu LL. Systematic review of barriers to the recruitment of older patients with cancer onto clinical trials. J Clin Oncol 2005;23: 3112–24.

27. Wang S, Wong ML, Hamilton N, et al. Impact of age and comorbidity on non-small-cell lung cancer treatment in older veterans. J Clin Oncol 2012;30:1447–55.

28. Partridge JS, Harari D, Dhesi JK. Frailty in the older surgical patient: a review. Age Aging 2012;41:142–7.

29. Sündermann S, Dademasch A, Praetorius J, et al. Comprehensive assessment of frailty for elderly high-risk patients undergoing cardiac surgery. Eur J Cardiothorac Surg 2011;39:33–7.

30. Afialo J, Mottillo S, Eisenberg MJ, et al. Addition of frailty and disability to cardiac surgery risk scores identifies elderly patients at high risk of mortality or major morbidity. Circ Cardiovasc Qual Outcomes 2012;5:222–8.

31. Yoshimura H. Quality of life (QOL) versus curability for lung cancer surgery. Ann Thorac Cardiovasc Surg 2001;7:127–32.

32. Ware JE, Sherbourne CD. The MOS 36-Item Short-Form Health Survey (SF-36). I. Conceptual framework and item selection. Med Care 1992;30:473–83.

33. Aaronson NK, Ahmedzai S, Bergman B, et al. The European Organization for Research and Treatment of Cancer QLQ-C30: a quality of life instrument for use in international clinical trials of oncology. J Natl Cancer Inst 1993;85:365–77.

34. Mangione CM, Goldman L, Orav J, et al. Health-related quality of life after elective surgery: measurement of longitudinal changes. J Gen Intern Med 1997;12:686–97.

35. Chen JC, Johnstone SA. Quality of life after lung cancer surgery: a forgotten outcome measure. Chest 2002;122:4–5.

36. Bergman B, Aaronson NK, Ahmedzai S, et al. The EORTC QLQ-LC13: a modular supplement to the EORTC Core Quality of Life Questionnaire (QLQ-C30) for use in lung cancer clinical trials. Eur J Cancer 1994;30:635–42.

37. Saad ED, Adamowicz K, Katz A, et al. Assessment of quality of life in advanced non-small-cell lung cancer: an overview of recent randomized trials. Cancer Treat Rev 2012;38(6):807–14 [Epub 2012 Mar 23].

38. Allison PJ, Locker D, Feine JS. Quality of life: a dynamic construct. Soc Sci Med 1997;45:221–30.

39. Li WW, Lee TW, Yim AP. Quality of life after lung cancer resection. Thorac Surg Clin 2004;14:353–65.

40. Sloan JA, de Andrade M, Decker P, et al. Genetic variations and patient-reported quality of life among patients with lung cancer. J Clin Oncol 2012;30:1699–704.

41. Zieren HU, Müller JM, Hamberger U, et al. Quality of life after surgical therapy of bronchogenic carcinoma. Eur J Cardiothorac Surg 1996;10:233–7.

42. Sartipy U. Prospective population-based study comparing quality of life after pneumonectomy and lobectomy. Eur J Cardiothorac Surg 2009;26:1069–74.

43. Schulte T, Schniewind B, Dohrmann P, et al. The extent of lung parenchyma resection significantly impacts long-term quality of life in patients with non-small cell lung cancer. Chest 2009;135:322–9.

44. Balduyck B, Hendriks J, Lauwers P, et al. Quality of life evolution after lung cancer surgery in septuagenarians: a prospective study. Eur J Cardiothorac Surg 2009;35:1070–5.

45. Handy JR, Asaph JW, Skokan L, et al. What happens to patients undergoing lung cancer surgery? Outcomes and quality of life before and after surgery. Chest 2002;122:21–30.

46. Pompili C, Brunelli A, Refai M, et al. Does chronic obstructive pulmonary disease affect postoperative quality of life in patients undergoing lobectomy for lung cancer? a case-matched study. Eur J Cardiothorac Surg 2010;37:525–30.

47. Brunelli A, Socci L, Refai M, et al. Quality of life before and after major lung resection for lung cancer: a prospective follow-up analysis. Ann Thorac Surg 2007;84:410–6.

48. O'Connell JB, Maggard MA, Ko CY. Cancer-directed surgery for localized disease: decreased use in the elderly. Ann Surg Oncol 2004;11:962–9.

49. Reeve BB, Potosky AL, Smith AW, et al. Impact of cancer on health-related quality of life of older Americans. J Natl Cancer Inst 2009;101:860–8.

50. Chambers A, Routeledge T, Pilling J. In elderly patients with lung cancer is resection justified in terms of morbidity, mortality and residual quality of life? Interact Cardiovasc Thorac Surg 2010;10:1015–21.

51. Salati M, Brunelli A, Xiumè F, et al. Quality of life in the elderly after major lung resection for lung cancer. Interact Cardiovasc Thorac Surg 2009;8:79–83.

52. Schulte T, Schniewind B, Walter J, et al. Age-related impairment of quality of life after lung resection for non-small cell lung cancer. Lung Cancer 2010;68:115–20.

53. Burfeind WR, Tong BC, O'Branski E, et al. Quality of life outcomes are equivalent after lobectomy in the elderly. J Thorac Cardiovasc Surg 2008;136:597–604.

54. Ferguson MK, Parma CM, Celauro AD, et al. Quality of life and mood in older patients after lung resection. Ann Thorac Surg 2009;87:1007–13.

55. Yang P, Cheville AL, Wampfler JA, et al. Quality of life and symptom burden among long-term cancer survivors. J Thorac Oncol 2012;7:64–70.

56. Das M, Abdelmaksoud MH, Loo BW, et al. Alternatives to surgery for early stage non-small cell lung cancer—ready for prime time? Curr Treat Options Oncol 2010;11:24–35.

57. Donington JS, Blasberg JD. Management of early stage non-small cell lung cancer in high-risk patients. Thorac Surg Clin 2012;22:55–65.

58. Ginsberg RJ, Rubinstein LV. Lung Cancer Study Group. Randomized trial of lobectomy versus limited resection for T1 N0 non-small cell lung cancer. Ann Thorac Surg 1995;60:615–23.

59. Balduyck B, Hendriks J, Lauwers P, et al. Quality of life evolution after lung cancer surgery: a prospective study in 100 patients. Lung Cancer 2007;56:423–31.

60. Kates M, Swanson S, Wisnivesky JP. Survival following lobectomy and limited resection for the treatment of stage I non-small cell lung cancer ≤1 cm in size: a review of SEER data. Chest 2011;139:491–6.

61. McKenna RJ, Mahtabifard A, Yap J, et al. Wedge resection and brachytherapy for lung cancer in patients with poor pulmonary function. Ann Thorac Surg 2008;85:S733–6.

62. Fernando HC, Landreneau RJ, Mandrekar SJ, et al. The impact of adjuvant brachytherapy with sublobar resection on pulmonary function and dyspnea in high-risk patients with operable disease: preliminary results from the American College of Surgeons Oncology Group Z4032 Trial. J Thorac Cardiovasc Surg 2011;142:554–62.

63. Li WW, Lee TW, Lam SS, et al. Quality of life following lung cancer resection: video-assisted thoracic surgery vs. thoracotomy. Chest 2002;122:584–9.

64. Paul S, Altorki NK, Sheng S, et al. Thoracoscopic lobectomy is associated with lower morbidity than open lobectomy: a propensity-matched analysis from the STS database. J Thorac Cardiovasc Surg 2010;139:366–78.

65. Berry MF, Onaitis M, Tong BC, et al. A model for morbidity after lung resection in octogenarians. Eur J Cardiothorac Surg 2011;39:989–94.

66. Fernando HC, Schuchert M, Landreneau R, et al. Approaching the high-risk patient: sublobar resection, stereotactic body radiation therapy, or radiofrequency ablation. Ann Thorac Surg 2010;89:S2123–7.

67. Widder J, Postmus D, Ubbels JF, et al. Survival and quality of life after stereotactic or 3D-conformal radiotherapy for inoperable early-stage lung cancer. Int J Radiat Oncol Biol Phys 2011;81:e291–7.

68. Onishi H, Shirato H, Nagata Y, et al. Stereotactic body radiotherapy (SBRT) for operable stage I non-small cell lung cancer: can SBRT be comparable to surgery? Int J Radiat Oncol Biol Phys 2011;81:1352–8.

69. Crabtree TD, Denlinger CE, Meyers BF, et al. Stereotactic body radiation therapy versus surgical resection for stage I non-small cell lung cancer. J Thorac Cardiovasc Surg 2010;140:377–86.

70. Abbas G, Pennathur A, Landreneau RJ, et al. Radiofrequency and microwave ablation of lung tumors. J Surg Oncol 2009;100:645–50.

71. Lencioni R, Crocetti L, Cioni R, et al. Response to radiofrequency ablation of pulmonary tumours: a prospective, intention-to-treat, multicentre clinical trial (the RAPTURE study). Lancet Oncol 2008;9: 621–8.

72. Kaplan RM, Feeny D, Revicki DA. Methods for assessing relative importance in preference based outcome measures. Qual Life Res 1993;2:467–75.

73. Brundage MD, Groome PA, Feldman-Stewart D, et al. Decision analysis in locally advanced non-small-cell lung Cancer: is it useful? J Clin Oncol 1997;15:873–83.

74. Cykert S, Kissling G, Hansen CJ. Patient preferences regarding possible outcomes of lung resection: what outcomes should preoperative evaluations target? Chest 2000;117:1551–9.

75. Dowie J, Wildman M. Choosing the surgical mortality threshold for high-risk patients with stage IA non-small cell lung cancer: insights from decision analysis. Thorax 2002;52:7–10.

76. Sher DJ, Wee JO, Punglia RS. Cost-effectiveness analysis of stereotactic body radiotherapy and radiofrequency ablation for medically-inoperable early-stage non-small cell lung cancer. Int J Radiat Oncol Biol Phys 2011;81:e767–74.

77. Puri V, Crabtree TD, Kymes S, et al. A comparison of surgical intervention and stereotactic body radiation therapy for stage I lung cancer in high-risk patients: a decision analysis. J Thorac Cardiovasc Surg 2012; 143:428–36.

78. Louie AV, Rodrigues G, Hannouf M, et al. Stereotactic body radiotherapy versus surgery for medically operable stage I non-small-cell lung cancer: a Markov model-based decision analysis. Int J Radiat Oncol Biol Phys 2011;81:964–73.

79. Cykert S. Risk acceptance and risk aversion: patients' perspectives on lung surgery. Thorac Surg Clin 2004;14:287–93.

80. Wang S, Krajbich I, Adolphs R, et al. The role of risk aversion in non-conscious decision making. Front Psychol 2012;3:50.

81. Epstein RM, Alper BS, Quill TE. Communicating evidence for participatory decision making. JAMA 2004;291:2359–66.

82. Davidoff AJ, Teng M, Seal B, et al. Chemotherapy and survival benefit in elderly patients with advanced non-small-cell lung cancer. J Clin Oncol 2010;28:2191–7.

83. Lara PN, Higdon R, Lim N, et al. Prospective evaluation of cancer clinical trial accrual patterns: identifying potential barriers to enrollment. J Clin Oncol 2001;19:1728–33.

Surviving the Intensive Care
Residual Physical, Cognitive, and Emotional Dysfunction

Christina Jones, BSc, MPhil, PhD, CSci, MBACP, DipH[a,b,*]

KEYWORDS

- Physical weakness • Cognitive problems • PTSD • Anxiety • Depression

KEY POINTS

- Patients recovering from critical illness may suffer from physical, psychological, and cognitive problems that have a negative impact on their health related quality of life.
- To ensure that patients return to as close as possible to their previous physical and mental health, their rehabilitation needs should be assessed and an appropriate program started.
- Early mobilization and physical rehabilitation while the patient is still in the intensive care unit (ICU) have been shown to improve physical functioning.
- Manualized rehabilitation after discharge from the ICU improves physical functioning, and ICU diaries reduce the incidence of posttraumatic stress disorder, depression, and anxiety.
- It is important to assess the rehabilitation needs of patients and target physiotherapy and counseling resources at those patients with the greatest need.

INTRODUCTION

When patients are discharged from critical care, their recovery may be uncertain and those who have had a prolonged stay in the intensive care unit (ICU) are likely to have the greatest physical rehabilitation needs as a result of gross muscle mass loss and joint stiffness. Some patients who have only a relatively short ICU stay of less than 5 days may still experience psychological problems such as anxiety, depression, or posttraumatic stress disorder (PTSD), but, regardless of their length of ICU stay, some patients make an uneventful recovery. Therefore, it is important to target rehabilitation resources where they are needed the most. Prolonged physical recovery and psychological problems resulting from critical illness have been described in several studies.[1–3]

PHYSICAL PROBLEMS

Muscle wasting and weakness following critical illness are common,[4] may take months to recover from, and are more likely with lengthy ICU stays and longer hours of ventilation.[5] Paired muscle biopsy studies have shown losses of up to 3% per day for type 1 muscle fibers and 4% per day for type 2 muscle fibers.[6] In addition, the protein loss from muscle during multiorgan failure can reach 2% per day.[7] Different patient factors can be used to identify patients in need of physical rehabilitation depending on a particular activity. For walking downstairs, which requires good quadriceps strength, age and length of ICU stay are predictors of difficulty, whereas for walking outside on uneven ground, premorbid health also has a negative impact, in addition to age and length of stay.[5] In

[a] Ward 4E (Critical Care), Warrington Road, Whiston Hospital, Prescot, L35 5DR United Kingdom;
[b] Department of Musculoskeletal Biology, Institute of Aging and Chronic Disease, University of Liverpool, Liverpool, L69 3GE United Kingdom
* Ward 4E (Critical Care), Warrington Road, Whiston Hospital, Prescot, L35 5DR UK.
E-mail address: christina.jones@sthk.nhs.uk

Thorac Surg Clin 22 (2012) 509–516
http://dx.doi.org/10.1016/j.thorsurg.2012.07.003
1547-4127/12/$ – see front matter © 2012 Elsevier Inc. All rights reserved.

addition to muscle mass losses resulting in muscle weakness, critical illness motor and sensory polyneuropathy can complicate and significantly lengthen the physical recovery picture.[8]

PSYCHOLOGICAL SEQUELAE

Psychological problems, such as anxiety, depression, PTSD, agoraphobia, panic attacks, and hospital phobia, can complicate recovery, negatively affect the patient's health-related quality of life (HRQOL), and increase the difficulty of any future medical care.[9,10] Traumatic memories from the patient's ICU stay, such as delusional memories of staff trying to kill the patient, can precipitate the development of PTSD.[3] Such memories are usually described by patients as being very vivid and realistic and therefore can be very frightening to recall; these memories may be replayed as recurrent nightmares or flashbacks once the patient has left the ICU. One study showed that approximately 10% of patients recovering from critical illness develop new-onset PTSD.[3] Patients with the full diagnosis of PTSD and for whom no help is offered may become socially isolated and alienated from their family and others. In addition, they may not return to their normal life because they avoid doing things that trigger an exacerbation of their symptoms. Alcohol and drug abuse can occur in this patient group in an effort to self-medicate to control their symptoms.[3] A systematic review of PTSD studies in ICU patients showed a median point prevalence of clinician-diagnosed PTSD of 19%.[11] In the included studies, consistent predictors of PTSD developing after an ICU stay were previous psychopathology, high-dose ICU benzodiazepine administration, and memories of frightening and/or psychotic experiences in ICU. The review showed that the development of PTSD following critical illness was associated with substantially lower HRQOL.

Such psychological problems can affect physical rehabilitation because it may be difficult for the patient to leave the house on his or her own. In addition, ongoing care of any chronic medical problems may be negatively affected, especially when the patient becomes panic stricken when attending the hospital. Recognition of psychological problems such as PTSD is very important, and an appropriate referral pathway for psychological treatment should be in place to enable timely therapy.

COGNITIVE DEFICITS

Recently, there has been recognition of the impact of cognitive problems that can occur following critical illness and how patients can find these issues distressing.[12] One particular group of patients, those recovering from adult respiratory distress syndrome, have been studied in particular, and at the 2-year follow-up point after discharge from ICU, 47% have been shown to still have cognitive impairment.[13] Deficits in memory, decision making, and attention have been shown, with the defects principally involving executive function. The executive system controls and manages other cognitive processes. This concept is used to describe a collection of brain processes responsible for planning, cognitive flexibility, abstract thinking, rule acquisition, initiating appropriate action, suppressing inappropriate actions, and selecting relevant sensory information. Deficits in executive functioning have also been demonstrated in general ICU patients at 3, 6, and 9 months after ICU discharge.[14–16] Increased absent-mindedness has also been reported in post-ICU patients.[12] Many patients with such problems gradually recover by themselves during the year following their illness, but they still require information about this so that they are prepared to be patient with the recovery process.

Informational Needs

During the patients' stay in the ICU and hospital and when they go home, their needs for information gradually change. While in the ICU, most patients are too ill to take in information and retain it. But transfer to the general ward can be a period of profound anxiety and worry about the future. Information should be given about their illness, speed of recovery, and possible psychological effects. In patients with adult respiratory distress syndrome who are preparing for hospital discharge, information is needed about their recovery and rehabilitation process.[17] The fragmented nature of many ICU patients' recall of their illness also means that their understanding of their illness is very poor.[18] The lack of such an autobiographic memory means that patients find it hard to understand why they feel so weak and easily tired. It also puts them at odds with their family, who have very clear memories of the ICU stay and may try to overprotect the patient, interfering with physical rehabilitation.

PHYSICAL REHABILITATION

Specific therapies to aid rehabilitation from critical illness have started to be examined, both while the patient is in the ICU and during the early part of their convalescence. Studies of patients in the ICU have looked at the benefits of early mobilization and physical rehabilitation. One study showed that simply mobilizing patients early in their time in the ICU reduced their length of stay in critical care and shortened their hospital stay.[19] Physical rehabilitation started as soon as possible while the patient is still critically ill resulted in an increase in the distance the patient walked in 6 minutes, improved isometric quadriceps force, and improved well-being at hospital discharge.[20] A third randomized controlled trial (RCT) with a graded intervention depending on the patients' condition, starting with passive exercises with sedated patients, progressing to active assisted and then active independent exercises, compared this with clinician-ordered therapy as the control. This study found that the intervention patients were more likely to return to independent functional status at hospital discharge compared with the control group.[21] There was also a reduction in delirium in the intervention patients and more ventilator-free days.

Some evidence exists for the efficacy of rehabilitation after discharge from intensive care. The provision of the *ICU Recovery Manual*, which is a manualized, 6-week multimodal rehabilitation program including exercises, psychological advice, and information on the after-effects of critical illness, has been shown in an RCT to accelerate physical recovery at 6 months after ICU discharge and had some effect on depression at 2 months.[22] The manual is explained to the patient and a family member if available by a nurse or physiotherapist about 1 week after ICU discharge, and the first set of exercises are chosen together. After this, the program is designed to be self-directed and so allows the patient to take back control of his or her recovery and enable the patient to devise his or her own exercise program to regain strength. A cohort of the patients from 1 center of the original multicenter study also recorded their smoking habits, because the manual contains smoking cessation advice. The intervention patients in this cohort showed a significantly increased rate of smoking cessation at both 2 and 6 months compared with the control group.[23]

Outpatient classes for convalescent critical care patients have been devised based on circuit training with the patient moving from 1 exercise station to the next, targeting different muscle groups. The Program of Enhanced Physiotherapy & Structured Exercise (PEPSE) consists of one 2-hour outpatient class combined with 2 home-based sessions per week for 6 weeks. A small, non-randomized pilot of PEPSE with 8 patients showed an improvement in the distance the patient walked in 6 minutes and a reduction in anxiety and depression scores.[24] In contrast, a recent RCT of an individualized 8-week home-based physical rehabilitation program did not show any improvement in physical function scores on the Short Form-36 or the distance walked on the 6-minute walk test between the intervention and control groups.[25] The cohort of patients included in the study had a median length of stay in ICU of 6 days compared with those in the *ICU Recovery Manual* study,[22] where the median stay was 14 days. Therefore, it could be expected that there would be significantly more muscle weakness and wasting and a longer recovery time. Because early mobilization and physical rehabilitation while the patient is in the ICU are being more widely adopted, it may be the number of patients who require outpatient physiotherapy is being reduced.

Those patients who develop a critical illness polyneuromyopathy during their ICU stay may benefit from neurorehabilitation. An Italian study looked at the degree of recovery achieved by patients with critical illness polyneuromyopathy and found that they had prolonged stays in neurorehabilitation, with a mean 76.2 days. The patients made good physical recovery in this setting.[26]

PSYCHOLOGICAL REHABILITATION
ICU Diaries

ICU diaries written by critical care nursing staff and the patients' family have been used since the 1980s, and their adoption is increasing worldwide.[27] They have been shown to help patients come to terms with their critical illness.[28] They are used in around half of the ICUs in Norway,[29] about a third of Danish ICUs,[30] and 75% of Swedish ICUs,[31] and their use is gradually increasing in the United Kingdom, Italy, and Portugal.[32] Diaries have been used for systematic follow-up, when patients try to understand what memories they have from the ICU,[33,34] and they seem to be helpful for both the patient and their families.[27,35,36] They can fill in the gaps in patients' memories of their illness. It has also been shown that diaries can be seen as showing the presence of the nurses to the patient and are a source of comfort and encouragement and a method of giving hope.[35] When trying to reconstruct a critical care illness experience for a patient, a diary gives a much more comprehensive picture of their stay than do the hospital records.[37]

The impact on the patients' psychological recovery of receiving an ICU diary has been tested in 2 RCTs. A small study (N = 36) of the effect of diaries on the incidence of anxiety and depression after critical illness showed a reduction in symptom scores for those patients receiving a written diary.[38] A larger RCT, in which 352 patients completed the 3-month follow-up, looked at the impact of receiving an ICU diary on the development of new-onset PTSD. These diaries were written by the nurses and the patients' families during their ICU stay and were a day-to-day account of their critical illness with photographs taken at points of change. A set of guidelines for writing diaries were used to help make the way they were written at each study center as consistent as possible across the 12 sites. The intervention patients received their diary at 1 month after ICU discharge, whereas the control patients waited until they had completed the final questionnaires at 3 months. There was a reduced incidence of new-onset PTSD at 3 months after ICU discharge in the intervention patients (5%) compared with the control group (13.1%) ($P = .03$).[39] The effect was most noticeable in those patients with high levels of PTSD symptoms at the point of receiving the diary. This suggests that the patients were using the diary to help themselves cope with the PTSD symptoms. One patient in the study reported that she took out her diary each time she had a flashback of a delusional memory she had of being taken out of a fire by firemen to read what really happened, which was that she was taken to the theater while still ventilated but not sedated.

COUNSELING AND PSYCHOTHERAPY

Specialist psychological services following critical illness are not generally available across Europe (personal communication). There are a few centers of excellence in the United Kingdom where such a service is offered, but other ICU patients and their families have to cope as best they can. In the United Kingdom, the National Institute of Clinical Excellence[40–42] has produced several treatment guidelines for anxiety, depression, and PTSD (**Box 1** for core tenets of guidelines). Of the core tenets, having a watch-and-wait approach for those patients who are coping with their symptoms is important and it gives patients space to see if they can use their normal coping strategies to come to terms with their experience. However, the patients should be reassessed at appropriate intervals to ensure that their symptoms are settling; if this is not happening, then they should be offered therapy. Those with high levels of symptoms at the first assessment that are having a detrimental effect on the patient's everyday functioning should be offered therapy immediately. Psychoactive medication should only be offered when patients do not feel able to engage in therapy.

Common themes expressed by patients undergoing counseling are trying to make sense of what happened in the ICU; coming to terms with

---

Box 1
Core tenet of National Institute of Clinical Excellence treatment guidelines for anxiety, depression, and PTSD

1. Need for assessment in high-risk groups, such as critical care patients
2. That an appropriate and timely referral should be made when symptom levels are high and interfering with everyday activities
3. That there should be a watch-and-wait approach for those patients with low symptom levels with a reassessment of symptoms at appropriate intervals
4. Advise that psychoactive medication should only be used if patients do not engage in psychotherapy

Data from Refs.[39–41]

---

physical changes, which in some cases may be permanent; and coping with distressing flashbacks or nightmares.[43] The National Institute of Clinical Excellence guideline[41] for the treatment of PTSD supports the use of both eye movement desensitization and reprocessing (EMDR) and cognitive-behavioral therapy (CBT). EMDR was developed to address psychological problems resulting from traumatic and unresolved life experiences. Past, present, and future aspects of these disturbing memories are examined by projecting them onto a cinema screen or watching them go by in a train window and then processed to reduce the distress the individual feels by bilateral stimulation of the brain through eye movements following the therapist's fingers from side to side.[43] Bilateral stimulation can also be provided with alternating tones in each ear or physical taps on the patient's hands or knees. CBT may include examining beliefs that are unhelpful or unrealistic, gradually facing activities that patients may have been avoided, and trying out new ways of reacting to stressful situations.

Clinical experience with counseling ICU patients[42] supports the use of EMDR and CBT. Their combined use results in most patients becoming nonsymptomatic or subclinical by the end of therapy[42] and the patients themselves report that they feel much better and can return to their normal activities and, importantly, engage with ongoing medical treatment when it is needed for chronic health conditions. PTSD in particular can stop patients from engaging ongoing medical treatment because the hospital becomes one of the places they avoid in an effort to reduce the triggering of intrusive memories from the ICU.

PATIENT AND FAMILY SUPPORT GROUPS

Support groups for recovering ICU patients and their families are becoming increasingly popular in the United Kingdom. The original model in the 1990s was led by the health care staff and required considerable staff resources to send out invitations and moderate the sessions.[44] It is necessary to use a meeting room away from the hospital because of the possible difficulty some patients will experience returning there. A more recent model is that followed by ICUsteps (a support group Web site that can be found at www.icusteps.org),[45] originally set up in Milton Keynes, UK, using patient and relative volunteers to help run the support group and raise funds.[46] This is a drop-in service meeting in the evening for 2 hours every 6 weeks at a meeting site away from the hospital where patients and their families can come, have coffee, and chat with the volunteers who are further along the road to recovery. This model is now being adopted more widely across the United Kingdom, with groups in Milton Keynes, London, Liverpool, Bristol, and South Tyneside. The support group allows patients and their families to normalize how they feel and share their experiences with others who immediately understand what they mean because they have been through it themselves.

Just speaking to other people helped, just to get it off your chest to speak to someone that's been through it (male patient 1).[46]

However, patients who already have PTSD may not be able to cope with the support group, so the ICUsteps model also includes a link on the Web site[45] for patients and families to email one of the volunteers or a staff member for advice. This means that the volunteer or staff member has to have a working knowledge of psychological problems such as PTSD so that they can give appropriate advice or refer for further assessment.

COGNITIVE REHABILITATION

Only a single pilot study has been performed so far on cognitive rehabilitation following critical illness, which involved 21 patients. The rehabilitation program was tolerated well by the intervention patients, and at the 3-month follow-up, they showed improved cognitive executive functioning compared with the control group.[47] It is interesting that the treatment of PTSD in patient groups other than those recovering from critical illness has also been shown to improve executive function, which is affected adversely in this disorder. A study undertaking neuropsychological testing within 1 week of PTSD treatment onset and approximately 3 months later in 15 women showed moderate improvement in executive function.[48] A second study of resilience-orientated treatment for PTSD in US Army veterans also showed moderate improvements in executive function and memory.[49] These findings highlight that the recognition and treatment of PTSD in our patients are very

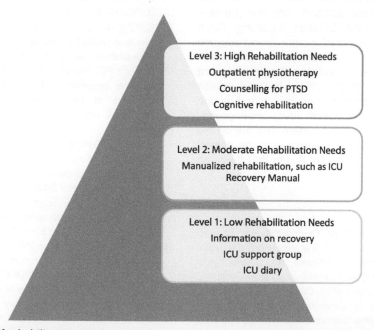

Level 3: High Rehabilitation Needs
Outpatient physiotherapy
Counselling for PTSD
Cognitive rehabilitation

Level 2: Moderate Rehabilitation Needs
Manualized rehabilitation, such as ICU Recovery Manual

Level 1: Low Rehabilitation Needs
Information on recovery
ICU support group
ICU diary

Fig. 1. Hierarchy of rehabilitation needs.

important and may have an additional effect on cognitive function that needs to be controlled for in future studies of cognitive dysfunction and rehabilitation, or it will be difficult to separate the effects.

SUMMARY

Many ICU patients are able to recover adequately without anything other than information about what to expect during their convalescence. However, for those who do have rehabilitation needs, whether physical, psychological, or cognitive, it is important for them to be assessed and appropriate help be given. Simple interventions such as ICU diaries can be provided at a small cost. Because they are written when the patient is still in the ICU, without knowing if a patient is going to have psychological problems during recovery, the diaries should be started for all ventilated patients staying 3 days and longer and offered to the patient after he or she leaves the ICU. The use of support groups such as ICUsteps is also a low-cost option; the initial work involved for health care staff is in bringing together the patient and family volunteers. Once this is done, the volunteers can start running the group. Support groups are a simple concept that is useful in helping patients and their families realize that they are not alone.

Those with greater rehabilitation needs may manage with a manualized approach such as the *ICU Recovery Manual*. This would leave the use of outpatient-based physiotherapy, cognitive rehabilitation, and counseling for PTSD and other conditions for those patients with the greatest needs (**Fig. 1** for rehabilitation hierarchy). Such a hierarchy ensures that scarce resources are concentrated where they can do the most good. What then becomes important is the development and validation of simple clinical tools to assess physical, psychological, and cognitive function so that patients' rehabilitation needs are appropriately recognized to identify where they are on the rehabilitation hierarchy. Patients must be helped to return to the best level of health that they can achieve.

REFERENCES

1. Angus DC, Musthafa AA, Clermont G, et al. Quality-adjusted survival in the first year after the acute respiratory distress syndrome. Am J Respir Crit Care Med 2001;163:1389–94.

2. Davidson TA, Caldwell ES, Curtis JR, et al. Reduced quality of life in survivors of acute respiratory distress syndrome compared with critically ill control patients. JAMA 1999;281:354–60.

3. Jones C, Backman C, Capuzzo M, et al. Precipitants of post-traumatic stress disorder following intensive care: a hypothesis generating study of diversity in care. Intensive Care Med 2007;33(6):978–85.

4. Herridge MS, Cheung AM, Tansey CM, et al. One-year outcomes in survivors of the acute respiratory distress syndrome. N Engl J Med 2003;348:683–93.

5. Jones C, Griffiths RD. Identifying post intensive care patients who may need physical rehabilitation. Clin Intensive Care 2000;11:35–8.

6. Helliwell TR, Wilkinson A, Griffiths RD, et al. Muscle fibre atrophy in critically ill patients is associated with the loss of myosin filaments and the presence of lysosomal enzymes and ubiquitin. Neuropathol Appl Neurobiol 1998;24:507–17.

7. Gamrin L, Andersson K, Hultman E, et al. Longitudinal changes of biochemical parameters in muscle during critical illness. Metabolism 1997;46:756–62.

8. Fletcher SN, Kennedy DD, Ghosh IR, et al. Persistent neuromuscular and neurophysiologic abnormalities in long-term survivors of prolonged critical illness. Crit Care Med 2003;31:1012–6.

9. Jones C, Griffiths RD. Patient and caregiver counselling after the intensive care unit: what are the needs and how should they be met? Curr Opin Crit Care 2007;13:503–50.

10. Jones C, Griffiths RD. Psychological Stress in adult ICU patients and relatives. In: Ridley S, editor. Critical care focus 12: the psychological challenges of intensive care. Oxford (United Kingdom): Blackwell Publishing; 2005. p. 39–49.

11. Davydow DS, Gifford JM, Desai SV, et al. Posttraumatic stress disorder in general intensive care unit survivors: a systematic review. Gen Hosp Psychiatry 2008;30(5):421–34.

12. Griffiths RD, Jones C. Delirium, cognitive dysfunction and posttraumatic stress disorder. Curr Opin Anaesthesiol 2007;20:124–9.

13. Hopkins RO, Weaver LK, Pope D, et al. Neurophysiological sequelae and impaired health status in survivors of severe acute respiratory distress syndrome. Am J Respir Crit Care Med 1999;160:50–6.

14. Jones C, Griffiths RD, Slater T, et al. Significant cognitive dysfunction in non-delirious patients identified during and persisting following critical illness. Intensive Care Med 2006;32(6):923–6.

15. Jackson JC, Hart RP, Gordon SM, et al. Six month neuropsychological outcome from medical intensive care unit patients. Crit Care Med 2003;31(4):1226–34.

16. Sukantarat KT, Burgess PW, Williamson RC, et al. Prolonged cognitive dysfunction in survivors of critical illness. Anaesthesia 2005;60:847–53.

17. Lee CM, Herridge MS, Matte A, et al. Education and support needs during recovery in acute respiratory distress syndrome survivors. Crit Care 2009;13(5):R153.

18. Griffiths RD, Jones C, Macmillan RR. Where is the harm in not knowing? Care after intensive care. Clin Intensive Care 1996;7:144–5.

19. Morris PE, Goad A, Thompson C. Early intensive care unit mobility therapy in the treatment of acute respiratory failure. Crit Care Med 2008;36:2238–43.

20. Burtin C, Clerckx B, Robbeets C, et al. Early exercise in critically ill patients enhances short-term functional recovery. Crit Care Med 2009;37(9):2499–505.

21. falseSchweickert WD, Pohlman MC, Pohlman AS, et al. Early physical and occupational therapy in mechanically ventilated, critically ill patients: a randomised controlled trial. Lancet 2009;373:1874–82.

22. Jones C, Skirrow P, Griffiths RD, et al. Rehabilitation after critical illness: a randomized, controlled trial. Crit Care Med 2003;31:2456–61.

23. Jones C, Griffiths RD, Skirrow P, et al. Smoking cessation through comprehensive critical care. Intensive Care Med 2001;27:1547–9.

24. McWilliams DJ, Atkinson D, Carter A. Feasibility and impact of a structured, exercise-based rehabilitation programme for intensive care survivors. Physiother Theory Pract 2009;25(8):566–71.

25. Elliott D, McKinley S, Alison J, et al. Health-related quality of life and physical recovery after a critical illness: a multi-centre randomised controlled trial of a home-based physical rehabilitation programme. Crit Care 2011;15:R142.

26. Intiso D, Amoruso L, Zarrelli M, et al. Long-term functional outcome and health status of patients with critical illness polyneuromyopathy. Acta Neurol Scand 2011;123(3):211–9.

27. ICU Diary Network. ICU diary. Available at: www.icu-diary.org. Accessed March 12, 2012.

28. Storli S, Lindseth A, Asplund K. A journey in quest of meaning: a hermeneutic-phenomenological study on living with memories from intensive care. Nurs Crit Care 2008;13(2):86–9.

29. Gjengedal E, Storli SL, Holme AN, et al. An act of caring: patient diaries in Norwegian intensive care units. Nurs Crit Care 2010;15(4):176–84.

30. Egerod I, Schwartz-Nielson KH, Hansen GM, et al. The extent and application of patient diaries in Danish ICUs in 2006. Nurs Crit Care 2007;12(3):159–67.

31. Åkerman E, Granberg-Axéll A, Ersson A, et al. Use and practice of the patient diaries in Swedish intensive care units: a national survey. Nurs Crit Care 2010;15(1):26–33.

32. Jones C, Bäckman C, Capuzzo M, et al. Intensive care diaries reduce new onset PTSD following critical illness: a randomised, controlled trial. Crit Care 2010;14:R168.

33. Bäckman C, Walther SM. The photo-diary and follow-up appointment on ICU: giving back time to patients and relatives. In: Ridley S, editor. Critical care focus 12: the psychological challenges of intensive care. Oxford (United Kingdom): Blackwell Publishing; 2001. p. 39–49.

34. Storli S, Lind R. The meaning of follow-up in intensive care: patients' perspective. Scand J Caring Sci 2009;23(1):45–56.

35. Robson W. An evaluation of patient diaries in intensive care. Connect: The World of Critical Care Nursing 2008;6(2):34–7.

36. Egerod I, Christensen D. Analysis of patient diaries in Danish ICUs: a narrative approach. Intensive Crit Care Nurs 2009;25(5):268–77.

37. Egerod I, Christensen D. A comparative study of ICU patients diaries vs. hospital charts. Qual Health Res 2010;22(10):1446–56.

38. Knowles RE, Tarrier N. Evaluation of the effect of prospective patient diaries on emotional well-being in intensive care unit survivors: a randomised control trial. Crit Care Med 2009;37:184–91.

39. National Institute of Clinical Excellence. Anxiety: management of anxiety (panic disorder, with or without agoraphobia, and generalised anxiety disorder) in adults in primary, secondary and community care. 2004. Available at: www.nice.org.uk/pdf/CG022NICEguideline.pdf. Accessed March 15, 2012.

40. National Institute of Clinical Excellence. Depression: management of depression in primary and secondary care: NICE guidance. 2004. Available at: www.nice.org.uk/CG023NICEguideline.pdf. Accessed March 15, 2012.

41. National Institute of Clinical Excellence. Post-traumatic stress disorder. The management of PTSD in adults and children in primary and secondary care. 2006. Available at: www.nice.org.uk/CG026NICEguideline.pdf. Accessed March 15, 2011.

42. Jones C, Hall S, Jackson S. Benchmarking a nurse-led ICU counselling initiative. Nurs Times 2008;104(38):32–4.

43. Shapiro F. EMDR as an integrative psychotherapy approach: experts of diverse orientations explore the paradigm prism. Washington, DC: American Psychological Association; 2002.

44. Jones C, Macmillan RR, Griffiths RD. Providing psychological support to patients after critical illness. Clin Intensive Care 1994;5(4):176–9.

45. ICUsteps. Available at: http://icusteps.org/. Accessed April 23, 2012.

46. Peskett M, Gibb P. Developing and setting up a patient and relatives intensive care support group. Nurs Crit Care 2009;14(1):4–10.

47. Jackson J, Ely EW, Morey MC, et al. Cognitive and physical rehabilitation of intensive care unit survivors: results of the RETURN randomized controlled pilot investigation. Crit Care Med 2012;40(4):1088–97.

48. Walter KH, Palmieri PA, Gunstad J. More than
    symptom reduction: changes in executive function
    over the course of PTSD treatment. J Trauma Stress
    2010;23(2):292–5.

49. Kent M, Davis MC, Stark SL, et al. A resilience-orien-
    tated treatment for posttraumatic stress disorder:
    results of a preliminary randomised clinical trial.
    J Trauma Stress 2011;24(5):591–5.

Psychosocial Issues Facing Lung Transplant Candidates, Recipients and Family Caregivers

Emily M. Rosenberger, BA[a], Mary Amanda Dew, PhD[b,c,d,e,*],
Andrea F. DiMartini, MD[b,f,g], Annette J. DeVito Dabbs, PhD, RN[h],
Roger D. Yusen, MD, MPH[i]

KEYWORDS

• Lung transplantation • Psychosocial factors • Psychological stressors • Quality of life

KEY POINTS

• Lung transplant candidates and recipients experience a range of psychosocial stressors throughout the transplant evaluation, waiting period, perioperative recovery, early years, and late-term years after transplantation.

• The lung transplantation process and its associated stressors affect a range of patient psychosocial outcomes, including global quality of life, physical functioning, psychiatric status, and adherence to the medical regimen.

• Lung recipients experience pre- to posttransplant gains in many psychosocial domains, although most gains plateau during the first posttransplant year at levels lower than those of the general population.

• Lung transplant candidates' and recipients' family caregivers are also exposed to stressors associated with the transplantation process, and their global quality of life and physical and emotional well-being may be affected as well.

• Transplant programs should incorporate evidence-based interventions to improve psychosocial outcomes and a combination of palliative and restorative care strategies that shift with patients' changing medical needs.

Funding support: Funded, in part, through the following grants from the National Institutes of Health: TL1 TR000145, R01 NR010711 and R01 HL083067.
Financial disclosures and/or conflicts of interest: The authors have nothing to disclose.
a Department of Clinical and Translational Science, School of Medicine, University of Pittsburgh, 3811 O'Hara Street, Pittsburgh, PA 15213, USA; b Department of Psychiatry, School of Medicine, University of Pittsburgh, 3811 O'Hara Street, Pittsburgh, PA 15213, USA; c Department of Psychology, University of Pittsburgh, 3811 O'Hara Street, Pittsburgh, PA 15213, USA; d Department of Epidemiology, University of Pittsburgh, 3811 O'Hara Street, Pittsburgh, PA 15213, USA; e Department of Biostatistics, University of Pittsburgh, 3811 O'Hara Street, Pittsburgh, PA 15213, USA; f Department Surgery, School of Medicine, University of Pittsburgh, 3811 O'Hara Street, Pittsburgh, PA 15213, USA; g Starzl Transplant Institute, University of Pittsburgh Medical Center, Pittsburgh, PA, USA; h Department of Acute & Tertiary Care, School of Nursing, University of Pittsburgh, 3500 Victoria Street, Pittsburgh, PA 15261, USA; i Division of Pulmonary and Critical Care Medicine, Washington University School of Medicine, 660 South Euclid Avenue, Campus Box 8052, St Louis, MO 63110, USA
* Corresponding author. Department of Psychiatry, School of Medicine, University of Pittsburgh, 3811 O'Hara Street, Pittsburgh, PA 15213.
E-mail address: dewma@upmc.edu

Thorac Surg Clin 22 (2012) 517–529
http://dx.doi.org/10.1016/j.thorsurg.2012.08.001
1547-4127/12/$ – see front matter © 2012 Elsevier Inc. All rights reserved.

Lung transplantation has become an accepted treatment for many individuals with severe lung disease.[1] It yields improvements in quality and/or quantity of life, depending on the underlying disease process leading to the transplant as well as many other pre- and posttransplant factors. Yet, transplant candidates and recipients experience a range of psychosocial issues that begin at the initiation of the transplant evaluation and continue throughout patients' wait for donor lungs, their perioperative recovery, and their long-term adjustment to posttransplant life. Psychosocial factors may comprise, be caused by, and result in changes to functional capacity, social roles and relationships, health maintenance behaviors, psychological status, perceptions of self, and life plans and goals. Quality of life has a strong association with these domains and their changes throughout the transplantation experience.

This article reviews the psychosocial factors implicated during the various phases of the lung transplantation experience. It will consider patients' perceptions of changes to quality of life and their reported well-being as they progress through each phase, with a focus on the following psychosocial domains: physical functioning, behavioral, psychological, and social. This article also highlights studies of interventions that aim to improve quality of care or reduce patient distress throughout the transplantation process. In addition, the authors address disease-specific differences in outcome, controversial issues in lung transplantation candidate selection, and palliative care for lung candidates and recipients. Lastly, they discuss some psychosocial effects of transplantation on patients' primary family caregivers, as caregivers play a major role in maintaining their loved ones' physical and mental health and also undergo significant exposure to the stressors of the transplantation experience.

EVALUATION FOR LUNG TRANSPLANTATION

Similar to other types of solid organ transplantation, the lung transplantation process begins in earnest as patients and their families begin to consider the idea of transplantation. Patients undergo a transplant evaluation that encompasses both medical and psychosocial realms. **Fig. 1** depicts examples of events and stressors that contribute to different phases of the transplantation experience, as well as some of the interventions that have demonstrated efficacy in reducing the impact of these stressors. Specific stressors associated with the evaluation include uncertainty about whether or not a transplant program will judge the potential transplant candidate as suitable for listing, fear of surgery, worry about changes to future life plans, financial strain, and conflicting feelings about treatment options.[2,3] Even participating in the transplant evaluation may cause distress and tension for some patients. Patients may be uncomfortable with the questions asked during the psychosocial portion of the evaluation because they are less familiar than those asked during the more routine medical portion of the evaluation. Patients may also be conflicted about whether revealing personal information that exposes their vulnerabilities may jeopardize their ability to present themselves favorably to maximize their chances of receiving a lung transplant.[3] Moreover, consideration of mental health in the transplant evaluation may engender stress due not only to the nature of the questions but also because the mental health professionals conducting the evaluation are focused on judging suitability for transplant rather than providing treatment.[4]

Ultimately, transplant candidates are confronted with the reality, and underlying stressor, that they risk opening themselves to the possibility of an arduous treatment that may never finally materialize. For some patients who have already accepted their progressive disease state, the hope of transplant and subsequent letdown may cause more distress than the management of the physical and psychological aspects of the disease itself. Patients' stage of acceptance of their need for a transplant, which often depends on the acuity of their disease, affects the level of distress patients experience while considering whether or not to undergo transplantation.[5] Patients with chronic, longstanding disease (eg, chronic obstructive pulmonary disease [COPD]) are more likely to have prepared themselves for the idea of a potentially long waiting period and the life changes that will ensue after the transplant than those patients with a more rapidly progressing illness and a shorter waiting time for transplant.

Patients with cystic fibrosis (CF)-associated lung disease are in a unique position with respect to accepting the idea of transplantation. Although disease counseling throughout their lifetime may have encouraged them to base life decisions on a projected rate of decline, transplantation represents a major change to their life timeline and simultaneously subjects them to stressors faced by all candidates about risks associated with the transplantation procedure.[6] High levels of anxiety and decisional conflict about being listed for transplantation commonly affect patients with CF. A recent study demonstrated the potential value of a decision aid for these patients. The investigators found that a paper- and internet-based tool that directly addressed CF-specific issues, offered in addition to standard pretransplant educational sessions,

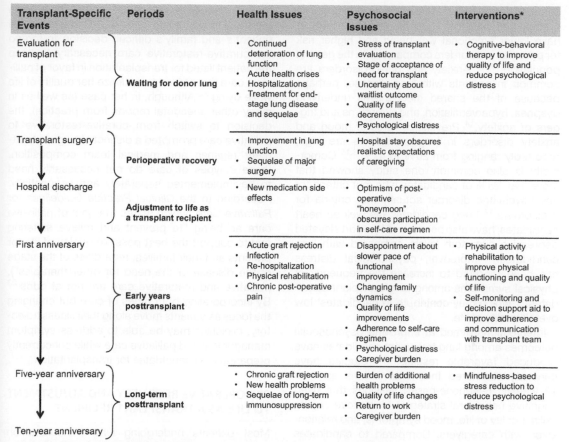

Transplant-Specific Events	Periods	Health Issues	Psychosocial Issues	Interventions*
Evaluation for transplant		• Continued deterioration of lung function	• Stress of transplant evaluation	• Cognitive-behavioral therapy to improve quality of life and reduce psychological distress
	Waiting for donor lung	• Acute health crises • Hospitalizations • Treatment for end-stage lung disease and sequelae	• Stage of acceptance of need for transplant • Uncertainty about waitlist outcome • Quality of life decrements • Psychological distress	
Transplant surgery	Perioperative recovery	• Improvement in lung function • Sequelae of major surgery	• Hospital stay obscures realistic expectations of caregiving	
Hospital discharge	Adjustment to life as a transplant recipient	• New medication side effects	• Optimism of postoperative "honeymoon" obscures participation in self-care regimen	
First anniversary	Early years posttransplant	• Acute graft rejection • Infection • Re-hospitalization • Physical rehabilitation • Chronic post-operative pain	• Disappointment about slower pace of functional improvement • Changing family dynamics • Quality of life improvements • Adherence to self-care regimen • Psychological distress • Caregiver burden	• Physical activity rehabilitation to improve physical functioning and quality of life • Self-monitoring and decision support aid to improve adherence and communication with transplant team
Five-year anniversary	Long-term posttransplant	• Chronic graft rejection • New health problems • Sequelae of long-term immunosuppression	• Burden of additional health problems • Quality of life changes • Return to work • Caregiver burden	• Mindfulness-based stress reduction to reduce psychological distress
Ten-year anniversary				

* Examples of interventions that have been tested at various time points along the transplant continuum

Fig. 1. Lung transplant timeline: examples of events and stressors that contribute to different phases of the transplantation experience as well as interventions that have demonstrated efficacy in reducing the impact of these stressors.

made patients' expectations of potential surgical and posttransplant complications more realistic and reduced their feelings of decisional conflict about being listed for transplant.[7] Similar decision aids might positively affect potential transplant candidates who may expect to experience quality but not quantity of life improvements from transplantation, including patients with COPD.

THE WAITING PERIOD FOR LUNG TRANSPLANTATION

Once listed as a candidate, patients and their families enter what may be the most stressful period of the entire transplantation experience. Candidates and their families must balance the reality that they may not survive to the point of transplantation with the desire to make plans for life after transplantation. Lung candidates have described feeling that they have no choice but to accept that they and their family members must simply put their lives on hold until after the transplant surgery.[8]

Transplant candidates in general experience persistent anxiety about when, if ever, the call will come that a donor organ has become available. In addition, they typically experience monotony and frustration about the physical functional limitations associated with advanced disease, especially if they require oxygen support, as do many lung candidates. Patients who live in geographically remote areas may need to relocate to undergo transplantation, which further disrupts a candidate's family and adds to the sense of feeling hostage to the waiting list. Throughout the waiting period, some candidates feel supported by interacting with transplant recipients who can provide hope and fellow candidates who can identify with their current stressors[5]; however, jealousy may arise if one candidate receives a transplant before another.[9]

The stressors associated with waiting for transplant have a cumulative effect on patients' generally poor quality of life. Lung candidates appear to have a lower quality of life than candidates for other types of transplantation,[10,11] likely because of their illness burden and physical impairments. They tend to have lower emotional well-being and higher risk for psychiatric disorders compared with the general population.[12–14] Anxiety and panic disorders are common in patients with lung disease, perhaps because of the shared mechanisms underlying dyspnea, hyperventilation, and symptoms and triggers of anxiety.[14] Prevalence rates of mood and anxiety disorders in lung candidates are high, reportedly ranging from 20% to 47%.[3,15] Comorbidity is also common: one study showed that more than 25% of candidates who met criteria for any psychiatric disorder actually met criteria for 2 disorders.[14] Lung candidates (as well as heart candidates) have also been found to report elevated depressive symptom levels compared with liver candidates.[16] Moreover, psychological distress has been reported to increase the frequency of physical symptoms among lung transplant candidates,[14] which may contribute to candidates' low overall quality of life.

Interventions aimed at improving psychosocial outcomes among lung transplant candidates have produced favorable results.[17–19] Studies have generally structured their interventions as 8 to 12 weekly, telephone-based sessions that used cognitive behavioral strategies to improve coping skills, quality of life, mood symptoms, and relationships with caregivers. Compared to candidates who participated in control conditions, which varied between usual care and health education sessions depending on the study, candidates who received an intervention reported higher quality of life, fewer depressive and anxiety symptoms, lower perceived stress, and higher optimism and perceived social support.

PALLIATIVE CARE PRETRANSPLANT

Although receiving no empirical evaluation to date, interventions that address symptom management, end-of-life care, and palliative care also have potential importance in this population. Patients, families, and their physicians may face difficult and complex decisions regarding the implementation of such strategies while they focus on the hope of eventual transplantation. However, the pace with which some individuals decompensate may drive the need to address end-of-life considerations and palliative care as part of their medical treatment. Among candidates with CF, studies have demonstrated that palliative care takes a secondary role to aggressive medical management that aims to sustain patients until transplantation[20,21]; as a result, CF candidates are often likely to die in the intensive care unit without ever

having discussed end-of-life wishes.[20] A case report of a candidate with COPD depicted the patient's and family's difficult decision to forego the curative-restorative care necessary to keep the patient listed for transplantation in favor of palliative care that strived to optimize her quality of life while dying.[22] Although, in her case (as well as in many other anecdotal reports from practice), the decision to switch from curative-restorative to palliative care prompted a distinct change in treatment regimen and medical team composition, these 2 types of care do not necessarily need to be implemented separately and sequentially. According to the *Clinical Practice Guidelines for Palliative Care* (which states the goal of palliative care as being "to prevent and relieve suffering and to support the best possible quality of life for patients and their families, regardless of the stage of the disease or the need for other therapies"), palliative and restorative care are not at odds.[23] By incorporating both types of care but changing the focus as patients move along their illness trajectory, clinicians may be able to address symptom management and palliative care while concurrently preparing lung candidates for transplantation.

PERIOPERATIVE RECOVERY AND ADJUSTMENT TO LIFE AS A TRANSPLANT RECIPIENT

Most patients undergoing lung transplantation experience a rapid change in health soon after transplant. Often, they transit quickly from life with minimal lung function and maximal anxiety before the transplant to a posttransplant honeymoon period characterized by feelings of high optimism and anticipation of steadily improving lung function.[24] Many patients and their families face hospital discharge buoyed by the success of transplant surgery and encouraged by early postoperative improvement in lung function.[2] In addition, many families may have welcomed the respite from caring for their lung recipient during the postoperative hospital stay and have thus begun to think about posttransplant life, sometimes prematurely, without the burdens of caregiving. Consequently, they may begin to set unrealistic expectations about the recovery process and long-term posttransplant life.

This posttransplant optimism may present a barrier to patients' and their families' participation in self-management after the transplant. Patient education efforts may stall, as patients may not see the need to carry out self-care activities important for preventing posttransplant complications.[2] A qualitative study of lung recipients described this initial phase as "naiveté"; after experiencing a positive postoperative experience and then beginning to see the normalization of pulmonary function tests and oxygen levels, many recipients felt immune to transplant-related complications.[24] Although health care providers instructed recipients about the high incidence of acute graft rejection during the early postoperative phase, these lung recipients tended to attribute symptoms to non-transplant-related causes and opted to call their primary care provider instead of their transplant team about emergent symptoms. Only after recipients had developed rejection did they and their families become more vigilant of symptoms of potential rejection. However, although this adjustment reduced patients' initial sense of denial about their posttransplant medical vulnerabilities, it also prompted feelings of guilt for thinking they were uniquely exempt from complications that affect nearly all lung recipients.

THE EARLY YEARS AFTER TRANSPLANT

As recipients progress farther from their transplant surgery, they become increasingly reliant on themselves and their families to manage day-to-day posttransplant care, mainly because of longer periods between follow-up clinic appointments. Despite this positive achievement, recipients may feel anxious on realizing that their contact with the transplant team is diminishing. Family dynamics often remain in flux during the early months after transplant. As patients' steep rate of recovery during the early postoperative period begins to plateau, the slower pace of functional improvement may be disheartening even though patients generally have higher levels of posttransplant functional ability and quality of life compared to their pretransplant levels. It often takes several years after transplant for patients and their families to fully adjust to the new range of stressors associated with life posttransplant and to accept that, with the transplant, they have traded one chronic disease for another. Studies have observed posttransplant adjustment in multiple areas of psychosocial outcomes, which are discussed in the following sections.

Global Quality of Life

The most significant improvements in quality of life from pre- to posttransplant tend to occur during the early posttransplant phase and remain stable for several years thereafter.[25–27] Although lung recipients' quality-of-life levels are typically lower than the general (nondiseased) population,[25,28] they show dramatic improvements in health-related quality of life[1,26,29,30] and feelings of well-being and life satisfaction[28,31] when compared with their pretransplant ratings of these outcomes. Nevertheless, their rate of improvement in quality

of life tends to be slower than that of heart recipients, for example, most likely because their physical recovery from surgery is more prolonged.[31] In addition, improvements in quality of life tend to plateau between 6 and 7 months after transplant,[27,31] with smaller gains observed thereafter.

Physical Functioning

Improvements in physical functioning show a slower trajectory of change than do recipients' perceptions of improvements in global quality of life. Whereas global quality of life has been shown to reach its plateau around 6 months posttransplant, physical functioning has been shown to improve throughout the first 2 years after transplant before leveling off.[32] Similar to global quality-of-life ratings, physical functional status posttransplant does not reach that of the general population.[33]

Interventions that aim to improve physical functioning represent an important part of comprehensive posttransplant rehabilitation, particularly because transplantation has not been shown to bring about the same gains in exercise capacity that it does in lung function.[34] Many transplant centers thus enroll or refer lung recipients to some form of exercise or pulmonary rehabilitation program. A review of 7 studies of aerobic and resistance exercise training programs for lung recipients showed that exercise training brought about improvements in maximal and functional exercise capacity, skeletal muscle function, and bone mineral density, all of which are impaired in lung recipients.[35] Moreover, exercise training improved health-related quality of life over the course of each program. Studies published since the aforementioned review demonstrated improvements in lung function, functional exercise capacity,[36] physical fitness indicators, blood pressure,[33] and exercise tolerance[37] among recipients who participated in exercise training. In studies that included a comparison group, greater improvements were seen in the intervention group relative to controls. Given the overall positive outcomes of empirically tested exercise training programs with varied structures, transplant centers have some flexibility around program location (eg, inpatient vs home-based) and program structure (eg, frequency, duration, and content of sessions).

Another important element of physical functional status, chronic postoperative pain, affects 18% to 49% of lung recipients during the first several years posttransplant.[38,39] One study identified the pretransplant diagnosis of emphysema as the strongest correlate of pain in lung recipients at least 3 months after transplant. Correlates of pain at this time point included older age, having had a single lung transplant, higher levels of depression symptoms, and lower health-related quality of life in areas other than pain.[38] Another study of lung recipients who had survived, on average, 3.5 years posttransplant showed that more than half of patients with chronic pain believed that it had a major impact on their quality of life and, depending on the intensity of the activity, reported pain to be a limiting factor in their daily social activities.[39]

Side effects of maintenance immunosuppression also factor into patients' overall physical functional status. These side effects range from transient to permanent, and they vary with respect to the distress they produce. Because lung recipients receive higher doses of immunosuppression medications than any other solid organ recipients, they tend to experience the most side effects.[40] A study of 287 lung recipients showed that the most common side effects were tremor, hirsutism, changed appearance, gastrointestinal complaints, and fragile skin, whereas the most common moderately-to-severely distressing side effects were gastrointestinal complaints, changed appearance, moon face, fragile skin, and muscle weakness (**Fig. 2**). A review of psychiatric considerations when treating transplant recipients in a critical care context noted that the most common neurotoxic side effects of immunosuppressants include tremors, headache, restlessness, insomnia, vivid dreams, photophobia, hyperesthesia, anxiety, and agitation, all of which affected 40% to 60% of those on immunosuppressive medication.[9] In addition to causing discomfort and pain, studies have demonstrated that these symptoms affect patients' adherence to their medication regimen.[41,42]

Posttransplant Adherence to the Medical Regimen

Lung recipients must follow a complex self-management regimen as part of their posttransplant care. Adherence to this regimen is particularly important for lung recipients because, relative to recipients of other solid organs, lung recipients have higher rates of infection and acute and chronic rejection.[43,44] The regimen includes taking immunosuppressants; monitoring spirometry, vital signs, weight, and symptoms; communicating effectively with the transplant care team; attending clinic appointments; getting regular blood work, pulmonary function testing, chest X-rays, and bronchoscopies; and following diet and exercise guidelines. One study found wide variability in lung recipients' adherence across these components of their regimen. Out of 178 recipients observed for the first 2 years after transplant, only 13% of recipients were nonadherent to immunosuppressants (based on a combination of self- and family caregiver-report).[43] In contrast, 26% were nonadherent to clinical appointments, 62% were nonadherent to required

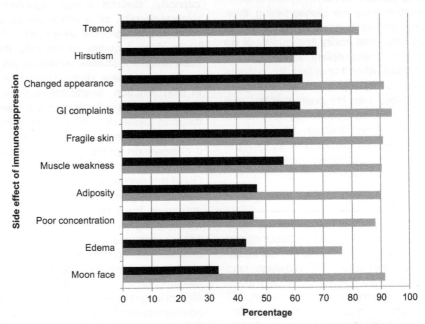

Fig. 2. Side effects of immunosuppression. Dark-shaded bars represent the prevalence of each symptom; light-shaded bars represent the percentage of those experiencing each symptom who found it moderately-to-severely distressing. (*Data from* Kugler C, Geyer S, Gottlieb J, et al. Symptom experience after lung transplantation: impact on quality of life and adherence. Clin Transplant 2007;21:590–6.)

spirometry, and 70% failed to monitor their blood pressure as required. In general, adherence declined over time.

University of Pittsburgh investigators recently developed an intervention that uses a handheld device called Pocket Personal Assistant for Tracking Health (Pocket PATH) to assist lung recipients with monitoring data related to their self-care behaviors and reporting potentially concerning values to the transplant team.[45] After 2 months of participation in a randomized controlled trial of Pocket PATH versus standard paper-and-pencil monitoring methods, recipients in the Pocket PATH group reported higher self-care agency, adherence to self-care behaviors, and quality of life than the other group. These findings support the need for further study of interventions to improve adherence to self-care behaviors, especially as recipients progress farther beyond the point of transplant. The University of Pittsburgh group is currently conducting a randomized trial to evaluate these long-term issues.

Aside from interventions that focus directly on adherence-related behaviors themselves, identification of risk factors for nonadherence after lung transplantation may allow for more targeted education of patients and their families. Risk factors identified to date include pretransplant nonadherence to medications, less social support, and lower conscientiousness[46]; more side effects from immunosuppressants[41]; and younger age.[47] Patients who considered themselves to have little influence over their health reported a higher rate of nonadherence to self-monitoring activities.[43] Similarly, patients with weaker beliefs in medications' ability to prevent rejection and stronger concerns about adverse effects of medication reported a higher rate of nonadherence to medication taking.[48] Although not yet used in lung transplant recipients, interventions that address patient knowledge about the role of self-management have improved adherence in nontransplant chronic disease populations.[49,50]

Psychiatric Status

Lung transplant recipients have reported prevalence rates of up to 30% for depression or anxiety disorders during the first year posttransplant, and these disorders are highly comorbid.[13,51] One study showed that despite similar rates of depression, posttraumatic stress disorder related to the transplant, and generalized anxiety disorder in lung and heart recipients, lung recipients had a significantly higher rate of panic disorder than heart recipients, with prevalence reaching 18% for lung recipients (relative to 8% in heart recipients).[13] Major risk factors for depression and/or anxiety included

having a history of these disorders, female gender, spending a longer time on the waiting list, having early posttransplant complications, and having poor caregiver support. Awareness of these predictors may allow clinicians to recognize patients at high risk for posttransplant psychiatric distress.

Despite the high rates of diagnosable psychiatric disorders, it is noteworthy that most patients do not experience such disorders.[12,13,25,28,51–53] Moreover, subclinical depression and anxiety symptoms tend to decline from pre- to posttransplant,[52] as recipients experience dramatic improvements in physical functioning and optimism about their recovery. Nevertheless, a significant minority may not show this improving pattern. In a study of lung, heart, liver, and kidney recipients, 40% showed declining levels of emotional well-being from pretransplant across the first 2 years posttransplant.[25] These individuals reported poorer pretransplant emotional well-being and a higher burden adhering to the posttransplant immunosuppressant regimen when compared with patients who had a more favorable pre- to posttransplant mental health profile. They may thus warrant additional support from the transplant team to avert a continued pattern of decline posttransplant.

The lung transplant literature lacks data regarding the impact of posttransplant psychiatric status on medical outcomes. A prospective study of 177 lung recipients found that depression and anxiety disorders did not predict mortality at up to 10 years posttransplant.[53] However, these disorders were associated with posttransplant morbidities, although in diverging directions. The study found that depression was associated with increased risk for bronchiolitis obliterans syndrome (BOS; the clinical correlate of chronic rejection), and lymphocytic bronchiolitis (the small airway disease that often precedes acute rejection), whereas anxiety was associated with decreased risk for graft loss and BOS. Adherence and frequency of screening (eg, pulmonary function tests and biopsies) did not mediate the relationship for either depression or anxiety.

THE LONG-TERM YEARS AFTER TRANSPLANT

After reaching plateaus in physical functioning and psychological adjustment to the transplant around the end of the first year posttransplant, lung transplant recipients tend to have more stability in medical and psychosocial outcomes during the subsequent years.[2,27] Recipients and their families shift their focus from preventing and caring for acute transplant-related complications to reestablishing normalcy in everyday life. Yet, the risk of medical complications does not disappear. Long-term survivors of lung transplantation develop chronic rejection and sequelae of prolonged immunosuppression (eg, diabetes,[2] renal failure,[54] osteoporosis,[55] malignancy,[56,57] neurologic complications, and opportunistic infections[58]). Some of these posttransplant complications, specifically, infections, rejections, and BOS, have been associated with reduced health-related quality of life[59] and an increased risk for anxiety and negative emotional well-being during the later posttransplant years.[60]

Indeed, the threat of BOS remains a predominant concern for recipients and their families, with impacts on many psychosocial domains. International transplant registry data suggest that BOS occurs in 49% of recipients by 5 years posttransplant and in 75% by 10 years.[61] Because BOS is largely unresponsive to treatment, mortality from BOS remains high among recipients who survive at least one year. One study reported frequent hospitalizations, emergency department visits, and intensive care unit admissions following the onset of chronic rejection.[62] The intense medical treatment required to manage BOS may explain the negative impact BOS has on multiple domains of psychosocial outcomes, including physical functional and emotional well-being.[27,63,64] Further, a qualitative study of family caregivers of lung recipients with chronic rejection showed that caregivers considered the incidence of BOS "inevitable" and were distraught by what they perceived as recipients' regression to their pretransplant state.[65]

Additional correlates of quality-of-life outcomes among long-term lung transplant survivors sometimes differ per outcome domain and time since transplant. Some studies showed a negative association between length of time since transplant and low quality of life in physical functioning domains in cohorts assessed at both 3 and 10 years posttransplant.[66,67] These recipients had lower quality-of-life scores than those of population norms and nontransplant chronic disease patients at 10 years. Conversely, another study found a positive association between length of time since transplant and mental health domains of quality of life, with quality-of-life scores equivalent to those of nontransplant populations at 10 years posttransplant.[67]

Predictors of low physical quality of life appear to differ according to time since transplant. In one study of recipients at 3 years posttransplant, some clinical events such as hospitalization predicted low physical quality of life.[66] Another study of recipients at 5 years posttransplant identified marital status and return to work as the strongest predictors.[27] At 10 years posttransplant, the strongest predictors of low physical quality of life were BOS, pretransplant physical quality of life, age, and gender.[63]

Predictors of psychosocial domains of quality of life differ from predictors of physical quality of life. Regarding psychological quality of life, BOS and pretransplant depression predicted posttransplant depression, whereas BOS and age predicted posttransplant anxiety, in a cohort of recipients at 10 years posttransplant.[63] In the social domain of quality of life, return to work has been considered one of the main indicators of success of transplantation, although only 28% to 39% of recipients have been found to be employed posttransplant.[27] Studies have shown that predictors of posttransplant employment include younger age, greater mobility, having had a previous occupation, having been off work for less than 2 years pretransplant, and having identified return to work as a main motivator for transplant.[68–70]

These findings underscore the need for psychosocial interventions that support recipients throughout the later-term posttransplant years. The only intervention study to date randomized solid organ recipients (including lung) to an 8-week long, weekly mindfulness-based stress reduction program, a peer-led health education program, or a standard care control.[71] One year after the end of the intervention, recipients who had received the intervention reported less anxiety and better sleep quality than recipients who had received the health education control and less depression and better sleep quality than recipients who had received the standard care control. Moreover, those who had received the intervention also reported increasing quality of life over the 8 weeks of the intervention. The study did not show differential effects of the intervention based on time since transplant.

CONTROVERSIAL POPULATIONS IN LUNG TRANSPLANTATION CANDIDATE SELECTION

Transplant programs strive to carefully select transplant candidates to optimize outcomes for patients and for the program. Such selectivity often leads to the exclusion of controversial patient populations. In many of these populations, psychosocial issues and outcomes may factor largely into the benefit they receive from transplantation, as is the case with older adults, or may complicate the decision to transplant them, as is the case with psychotic patients.

Older adults have demonstrated positive psychosocial outcomes after transplantation. A review of solid organ transplantation in older adults reported that older recipients have equivalent, and sometimes better, adherence, mental health outcomes, and quality of life relative to younger recipients.[72] Similarly, a study that compared lung recipients of various age groups showed that older recipients did not experience more posttransplant complications or worse hospital-related outcomes than younger recipients.[73] Moreover, the few studies that have considered the impact of age on posttransplant psychosocial outcomes have not found any predictive relationship.[72] Relative to the general population, however, older recipients reported higher rates of psychiatric disorders and lower rates of employment. Despite these favorable data regarding lung transplant outcomes in older adults, studies cannot fully adjust for the other factors that may lead transplant programs to screen out older candidates.

Transplant programs have traditionally considered patients with psychotic disorders to be questionable candidates for transplantation because of fears that the stress of transplantation or side effects from steroids will destabilize their psychotic disorder and subsequently cause nonadherence to the posttransplant regimen.[60] Across all organs, a survey of transplant programs' experiences with patients with psychotic disorders reported incidence rates of rejection and nonadherence to immunosuppressants that were consistent with rates seen in nonpsychotic organ recipients.[74] Specific to lung transplantation, one case report of a lung recipient with schizophrenia described favorable respiratory and psychiatric outcomes after lung transplantation, as well as consistent attendance at monthly visits to the psychiatric clinic.[75]

PALLIATIVE CARE POSTTRANSPLANT

The decision to initiate palliative care after transplant is complex because patients, families, and their clinicians may consider palliative care to conflict with the life-sustaining goals of transplantation. However, palliative care is not, by definition, end-of-life care; rather, it aims to optimize quality of life throughout patients' illness trajectory. In a study of palliative care referrals after lung transplantation, the misconception that palliative care is end-of-life care was endorsed by most transplant and palliative care clinicians as a barrier to initiating palliative care.[76] An additional barrier noted by transplant clinicians was uncertainty about patients' prognosis, which often prevented the initiation of palliative care until patients were ill enough to require stopping life-sustaining treatment. Moreover, the prospect of retransplantation makes the decision to stop aggressive treatment measures even more difficult for many patients and their families.[65] It may be ideal for palliative care and restorative care to proceed in parallel, with the focus of care shifting as patients' illness trajectory and treatment options change over time.

IMPACT ON CAREGIVERS OF TRANSPLANT RECIPIENTS

Family caregivers provide crucial supports for maintaining patients' physical and mental health throughout the transplantation process. During phases of the process in which patients may experience severe illness and disability, caregivers carry out practical activities that patients often take for granted in daily life. Exposure to the chronic stresses of transplantation may cause caregivers of both lung candidates and recipients to experience a lower quality of life than noncaregiving adults.[77] Moreover, up to 30% of caregivers for lung candidates reported clinically significant levels of depression and anxiety, both of which were associated with a higher perceived burden of caregiving.[78,79] Caregivers may feel confined and inconvenienced by having to be available to help their loved one at any time, and they may also feel disappointment that the illness has substantially changed their loved one.[77] One qualitative study determined that 30% of caregivers' daily activities during the first 6 months after transplant were related to supporting their loved one's health.[80] Although performing these activities can often be gratifying, adjusting to the changing family dynamics, household responsibilities, and job-related capacities associated with transplant may compound the discrete burdens of caregiving, as evidenced by caregivers reportedly spending less of their day in a positive mood than did the lung recipients for which they care.[80] At the same time, however, caregivers also reported positive outcomes of caregiving, such as discovering inner strength and support from others and realizing the important things in life.[77]

Interventions to improve caregivers' quality of life may have benefits for both patients' and caregivers' health. Evidence from nontransplant populations show that psychological interventions for caregivers of patients with a chronic illness may improve caregivers' mental health and coping skills.[81] The only such study in lung transplantation that evaluated the effect of a psychological intervention on caregivers' quality of life showed that caregivers of lung candidates who received the psychological therapy reported better quality of life, fewer mood disturbances, and higher social intimacy than caregivers of patients who did not receive the therapy.[82]

SUMMARY AND TREATMENT IMPLICATIONS

The process of lung transplantation brings with it a range of successes and stressors from the time a patient contemplates undergoing evaluation to the years beyond the transplant. Although transplantation may improve quality of life, physical functioning, and psychiatric status, not all patients experience the same degree of improvements; moreover, benefits do not always occur as quickly as many patients anticipate. Patients often expect that the transplant will restore their health and quality of life to a level comparable to levels before they ever became ill. Instead, adjustment to life after transplant often requires coming to terms with ongoing medical illness burden and continued reliance on caregivers. After experiencing improvements in pre- to posttransplant psychosocial status (eg, global quality of life, physical functioning, and mental health), patients' levels of psychosocial outcomes typically plateau and do not return to levels equivalent to the general population. Nevertheless, because patients may still experience dramatic pre- to posttransplant improvements in psychosocial status, clinicians should work with lung recipients and their families, particularly their caregivers, to find ways to sustain or increase those gains, such as by optimizing adherence, symptom management, and complication prevention.

Transplant programs could consider incorporating elements from the evidence-based interventions reviewed here into care of both candidates and recipients. Because most recipients and their families cite the waiting period as the most distressing part of the transplantation experience, pretransplant psychosocial interventions could include those that aim to ease the stresses related to the uncertainty of being on the waiting list while simultaneously managing a deteriorating condition. Immediately after transplant, although recipients and their families optimistically enjoy the successes of the surgery and patients' marked gains in physical functioning, interventions could focus on education about the risks of posttransplant complications and the importance of self-monitoring in order to involve patients in the prevention of infections and complications. During the years beyond the transplant, interventions could aim to improve quality of life (in both recipients and their caregivers), physical functioning, and adherence to the medical regimen. Although it is sometimes challenging to reconcile the treatment goals of patients, families, and the transplant team, evidence suggest that deliberate and preemptive integration of palliative care and restorative care maximizes quality of life over the course of the pre- to posttransplant illness trajectory; transplant programs could thus strive to offer palliative and restorative care in parallel.

To meet the broad needs of lung recipients and their families, clinicians must remain aware of the many psychosocial issues lung recipients face throughout the transplantation process. At the same time, clinicians should address the many psychosocial benefits recipients may experience, as a means of acknowledging progress and facilitating greater grains. An understanding of these psychosocial issues over the course of the transplantation timeline and an inclusion of approaches to improve various posttransplant issues based on evidence-based interventions may aid transplant programs in improving the care of their lung recipients.

REFERENCES

1. Yusen RD. Survival and quality of life of patients undergoing lung transplant. Clin Chest Med 2011; 32:253–64.
2. Dew MA, DiMartini AF, Kormos RL. Stress of organ transplantation. In: Fink G, editor. Encyclopedia of stress. 2nd edition. Oxford, UK: Academic Press (Elsevier); 2007. pp. 35–44.
3. Barbour KA, Blumenthal JA, Palmer SM. Psychosocial issues in the assessment and management of patients undergoing lung transplantation. Chest 2006;129:1367–74.
4. Olbrisch ME, Benedict SM, Ashe K, et al. Psychological assessment and care of organ transplant patients. J Consult Clin Psychol 2002;70:771–83.
5. Ivarsson B, Ekmehag B, Sjoberg T. Recently accepted for the waiting list for heart or lung transplantation - patients' experiences of information and support. Clin Transplant 2011;25:E664–71.
6. Adler FR, Aurora P, Barker DH, et al. Lung transplantation for cystic fibrosis. Proc Am Thorac Soc 2009; 6:619–33.
7. Vandemheen KL, O'Connor A, Bell SC, et al. Randomized trial of a decision aid for patients with cystic fibrosis considering lung transplantation. Am J Respir Crit Care Med 2009;180:761–8.
8. Naef R, Bournes DA. The lived experience of waiting: a Parse method study. Nurs Sci Q 2009;22:141–53.
9. DiMartini AF, Crone C, Fireman M, et al. Psychiatric aspects of organ transplantation in critical care. Crit Care Clin 2008;24:949–81.
10. Ortega T, Deulofeu R, Salamero P, et al. Health-related quality of life before and after a solid organ transplantation (kidney, liver, and lung) of four Catalonia hospitals. Transplant Proc 2009;41:2265–7.
11. Myaskovsky L, Dew MA, Switzer GE, et al. Quality of life and coping strategies among lung transplant candidates and their family caregivers. Soc Sci Med 2005;60:2321–32.
12. Dew MA, DiMartini AF. Psychological disorders and distress after adult cardiothoracic transplantation. J Cardiovasc Nurs 2005;20:S51–66.
13. Dew MA, DiMartini AF, DeVito Dabbs AJ, et al. Onset and risk factors for anxiety and depression during

the first two years after lung transplantation. Gen Hosp Psychiatry 2012;34:127–38.

14. Parekh PI, Blumenthal JA, Babyak MA, et al. Psychiatric disorder and quality of life in patients awaiting lung transplantation. Chest 2003;124(5):1682–8.

15. Erim Y, Beckmann M, Marggraf G, et al. Psychosomatic evaluation of patients awaiting lung transplantation. Transplant Proc 2009;41:2595–8.

16. Dobbels F, Vanhaecke J, Nevens F, et al. Liver versus cardiothoracic transplant candidates and their pretransplant psychosocial and behavioral risk profiles: good neighbors or complete strangers? Transpl Int 2007;20:1020–30.

17. Blumenthal JA, Babyak MA, Keefe FJ, et al. Telephone-based coping skills training for patients awaiting lung transplantation. J Consult Clin Psychol 2006;74:535–44.

18. Rodrigue JR, Baz MA, Widows MR, et al. A randomized evaluation of quality-of-life therapy with patients awaiting lung transplantation. Am J Transplant 2005;5:2425–32.

19. Napolitano MA, Babyak MA, Palmer S, et al. Effects of a telephone-based psychosocial intervention for patients awaiting lung transplantation. Chest 2002; 122:1176–84.

20. Sands D, Repetto T, Dupont LJ, et al. End of life care for patients with cystic fibrosis. J Cyst Fibros 2011; 10:S37–44.

21. Robinson WM. Palliative and end-of-life care in cystic fibrosis: what we know and what we need to know. Curr Opin Pulm Med 2009;15:621–5.

22. Janssen DJ, Spruit MA, Does JD, et al. End-of-life care in a COPD patient awaiting lung transplantation: a case report. BMC Palliat Care 2010;9:6.

23. National Consensus Project for Quality Palliative Care. Clinical Practice Guidelines for Palliative Care. 2nd edition. 2009. Available at http://www.nationalconsensusproject.org/guideline.pdf.

24. DeVito Dabbs A, Hoffman LA, Swigart V, et al. Striving for normalcy: symptoms and the threat of rejection after lung transplantation. Soc Sci Med 2004;59:1473–84.

25. Goetzmann L, Ruegg L, Stamm M, et al. Psychosocial profiles after transplantation: a 24-month follow-up of heart, lung, liver, kidney and allogeneic bone-marrow patients. Transplantation 2008;86:662–8.

26. Goetzmann L, Sarac N, Ambuhl P, et al. Psychological response and quality of life after transplantation: a comparison between heart, lung, liver and kidney recipients. Swiss Med Wkly 2008;138: 477–83.

27. Kugler C, Tegtbur U, Gottlieb J, et al. Health-related quality of life in long-term survivors after heart and lung transplantation: a prospective cohort study. Transplantation 2010;90:451–7.

28. Goetzmann L, Klaghofer R, Wagner-Huber R, et al. Quality of life and psychosocial situation before

and after a lung, liver or an allogeneic bone marrow transplant. Swiss Med Wkly 2006;136:281–90.

29. Yusen RD. Technology and outcomes assessment in lung transplantation. Proc Am Thorac Soc 2009;6: 128–36.

30. Eskander A, Waddell TK, Faughnan ME, et al. BODE index and quality of life in advanced chronic obstructive pulmonary disease before and after lung transplantation. J Heart Lung Transplant 2011; 30:1334–41.

31. Myaskovsky L, Dew MA, McNulty ML, et al. Trajectories of change in quality of life in 12-month survivors of lung or heart transplant. Am J Transplant 2006;6: 1939–47.

32. Bossenbroek L, ten Hacken NH, van der Bij W, et al. Cross-sectional assessment of daily physical activity in chronic obstructive pulmonary disease lung transplant patients. J Heart Lung Transplant 2009;28: 149–55.

33. Langer D, Gosselink R, Pitta F, et al. Physical activity in daily life 1 year after lung transplantation. J Heart Lung Transplant 2009;28:572–8.

34. Bartels MN, Armstrong HF, Gerardo RE, et al. Evaluation of pulmonary function and exercise performance by cardiopulmonary exercise testing before and after lung transplantation. Chest 2011;140(6): 1604–11.

35. Wickerson L, Mathur S, Brooks D. Exercise training after lung transplantation: a systematic review. J Heart Lung Transplant 2010;29:497–503.

36. Munro PE, Holland AE, Bailey M, et al. Pulmonary rehabilitation following lung transplantation. Transplant Proc 2009;41:292–5.

37. Vivodtzev I, Pison C, Guerrero K, et al. Benefits of home-based endurance training in lung transplant recipients. Respir Physiol Neurobiol 2011;177: 189–98.

38. Girard F, Chouinard P, Boudreault D, et al. Prevalence and impact of pain on the quality of life of lung transplant recipients: a prospective observational study. Chest 2006;130:1535–40.

39. Wildgaard K, Iversen M, Kehlet H. Chronic pain after lung transplantation: a nationwide study. Clin J Pain 2010;26:217–22.

40. Floreth T, Bhorade SM. Current trends in immunosuppression for lung transplantation. Semin Respir Crit Care Med 2010;31:172–8.

41. Kugler C, Geyer S, Gottlieb J, et al. Symptom experience after lung transplantation: impact on quality of life and adherence. Clin Transplant 2007;21:590–6.

42. Dobbels F, Vanhaecke J, Desmyttre A, et al. Prevalence and correlates of self-reported pretransplant nonadherence with medication in heart, liver, and lung transplant candidates. Transplantation 2005; 79:1588–95.

43. Dew MA, DiMartini AF, DeVito Dabbs A, et al. Adherence to the medical regimen during the first two

years after lung transplantation. Transplantation 2008;85:193–202.

44. De Geest S, Dobbels F, Fluri C, et al. Adherence to the therapeutic regimen in heart, lung, and heart-lung transplant recipients. J Cardiovasc Nurs 2005; 20:S88–98.

45. DeVito Dabbs A, Dew MA, Myers B, et al. Evaluation of a hand-held, computer-based intervention to promote early self-care behaviors after lung transplant. Clin Transplant 2009;23:537–45.

46. Dobbels F, Vanhaecke J, Dupont L, et al. Pretransplant predictors of posttransplant adherence and clinical outcome: an evidence base for pretransplant psychosocial screening. Transplantation 2009;87: 1497–504.

47. Bosma OH, Vermeulen KM, Verschurren EA, et al. Adherence to immunosuppression in adult lung transplant recipients: prevalence and risk factors. J Heart Lung Transplant 2011;30:1275–80.

48. Kung M, Koschwanez HE, Painter L, et al. Immunosuppressant nonadherence in heart, liver, and lung transplant patients: associations with medication beliefs and illness perceptions. Transplantation 2012;93: 958–63.

49. Bodenheimer T, Lorig K, Holman H, et al. Patient self-management of chronic disease in primary care. JAMA 2002;288:2469–75.

50. Holman H, Lorig K. Patient self-management: a key to effectiveness and efficiency in care of chronic disease. Public Health Rep 2004;119: 239–43.

51. Goetzmann L, Scheuer E, Naef R, et al. Psychosocial situation and physical health in 50 patients > 1 year after lung transplantation. Chest 2005;127: 166–70.

52. Vermeulen KM, Ouwens JP, van der Bij W, et al. Long-term quality of life in patients surviving at least 55 months after lung transplantation. Gen Hosp Psychiatry 2003;25:95–102.

53. Rosenberger EM, DiMartini AF, Toyoda Y, et al. Psychiatric predictors of 10-year outcomes after lung transplantation [abstract 374]. J Heart Lung Transplant 2012;31(4S):S132–3.

54. Mason DP, Solovera-Rozas M, Feng J, et al. Dialysis after lung transplantation: prevalence, risk factors and outcome. J Heart Lung Transplant 2007;26: 1155–62.

55. Kulak CA, Borba VZ, Kulak J Jr, et al. Transplantation osteoporosis. Arq Bras Endocrinol Metabol 2006;50: 783–92.

56. Anile M, Venuta F, Diso D, et al. Malignancies following lung transplantation. Transplant Proc 2007; 39:1983–4.

57. Kremer BE, Reshef R, Misleh JG, et al. Post-transplant lymphoproliferative disorder after lung transplantation: a review of 35 cases. J Heart Lung Transplant 2012;31:296–304.

58. Zivkovic SA, Jumaa M, Barisic N, et al. Neurologic complications following lung transplantation. J Neurol Sci 2009;280:90–3.

59. Kugler C, Tegtbur U, Gottlieb J, et al. Health-related quality of life in two hundred-eighty lung transplant recipients. J Heart Lung Transplant 2005;24:2262–8.

60. Rosenberger EM, Dew MA, Crone C, et al. Psychiatric disorders as risk factors for adverse medical outcomes after solid organ transplantation. Curr Opin Organ Transplant 2012;17:188–92.

61. Christie JD, Edwards LB, Kucheryavaya AY, et al. The Registry of the International Society for Heart and Lung Transplantation: twenty-eighth adult lung and heart-lung transplant report–2011. J Heart Lung Transplant 2011;30:1104–22.

62. Song MK, DeVito Dabbs A, Studer SM, et al. Course of illness after the onset of chronic rejection in lung transplant recipients. Am J Crit Care 2008;17:246–53.

63. Vermeulen KM, van der Bij W, Erasmus ME, et al. Long-term health-related quality of life after lung transplantation: different predictors for different dimensions. J Heart Lung Transplant 2007;26: 188–93.

64. van den Berg JW, Geertsma A, van der Bij W, et al. Bronchiolitis obliterans syndrome after lung transplantation and health-related quality of life. Am J Respir Crit Care Med 2000;161:1937–41.

65. Song MK, DeVito Dabbs A, Studer SM, et al. Exploring the meaning of chronic rejection after lung transplantation and its impact on clinical management and caregiving. J Pain Symptom Manage 2010;40:246–55.

66. Vasiliadis HM, Collet JP, Poirier C. Health-related quality-of-life determinants in lung transplantation. J Heart Lung Transplant 2006;25:226–33.

67. Rutherford RM, Fisher AJ, Hilton C, et al. Functional status and quality of life in patients surviving 10 years after lung transplantation. Am J Transplant 2005;5:1099–104.

68. Petrucci L, Ricotti S, Michelini I, et al. Return to work after thoracic organ transplantation in a clinically-stable population. Eur J Heart Fail 2007;9:1112–9.

69. Cicutto L, Braidy C, Moloney S, et al. Factors affecting attainment of paid employment after lung transplantation. J Heart Lung Transplant 2004;23: 481–6.

70. De Baere C, Delva D, Kloeck A, et al. Return to work and social participation: does type of organ transplantation matter? Transplantation 2010;89:1009–15.

71. Gross CR, Kreitzer MJ, Thomas W, et al. Mindfulness-based stress reduction for solid organ transplant recipients: a randomized controlled trial. Altern Ther Health Med 2010;6:30–8.

72. Abecassis MM, Bridges ND, Clancy CJ, et al. Solid organ transplantation in older adults: current status and future research. Am J Transplant 2012;12:2608–22.

73. Vadnerkar A, Toyoda Y, Crespo M, et al. Age-specific complications among lung transplant recipients 60 years and older. J Heart Lung Transplant 2011;30:273–81.

74. Coffman KL, Crone C. Rational guidelines for transplantation in patients with psychotic disorders. Curr Opin Organ Transplant 2002;7:385–8.

75. Okayasu H, Ozeki Y, Chida M, et al. Lung transplantation in a Japanese patient with schizophrenia from brain-dead donor. Gen Hosp Psychiatry April 26, 2012. [Epub ahead of print].

76. Song MK, DeVito Dabbs A, Studer SM, et al. Palliative care referrals after lung transplantation in major transplant centers in the United States. Crit Care Med 2009;37:1288–92.

77. Rodrigue JR, Baz MA. Waiting for lung transplantation: quality of life, mood, caregiving strain and benefit, and social intimacy of spouses. Clin Transplant 2007;21:722–7.

78. Goetzinger AM, Blumenthal JA, O'Hayer CV, et al. Stress and coping in caregivers of patients awaiting solid organ transplantation. Clin Transplant 2012;26:97–104.

79. Claar RL, Parekh PI, Palmer SM, et al. Emotional distress and quality of life in caregivers of patients awaiting lung transplant. J Psychosom Res 2005;59:1–6.

80. Xu J, Adeboyejo O, Wagley E, et al. Daily burdens of recipients and family caregivers after lung transplant. Prog Transplant 2012;22:41–7.

81. Selwood A, Johnston K, Katona C, et al. Systematic review of the effect of psychological interventions on family caregivers of people with dementia. J Affect Disord 2007;101:75–89.

82. Rodrigue JR, Widows MR, Baz MA. Caregivers of lung transplant candidates: do they benefit when the patient is receiving psychological services? Prog Transplant 2006;16:336–42.

The Patient-Surgeon Relationship in the Cyber Era
Communication and Information

J. Herman Blake, PhD[a], Mary Kay Schwemmer, JD[b],
Robert M. Sade, MD[c],*

KEYWORDS

- Patient-physician relationship • Information technology • Medical ethics • Bioethics • Telemedicine
- Telehealth • Malpractice

KEY POINTS

- A consistent pattern of increased use of the Internet by patients and their families has been well documented.
- Patients can benefit from telemedicine technologies in simple ways, such as advice from personal physicians by e-mail or through websites, and can also satisfy more demanding needs, such as long-distance consultation with specialists.
- Many studies of physicians' perceptions of electronic communication with patients have documented recognition of benefits as well as concerns about confidentiality, increased workload, inappropriate use, and medicolegal issues.

From Laennec's invention of the stethoscope in 1816 to the recently introduced Sapien transcatheter aortic valve replacement, the increasing complexity of health care technology has significantly affected the relationship between patients and physicians. Changing technology has increased accuracy and safety in health care, while also improving access to physicians through technologies that permit distance communications.

This article highlights some of the most important effects of telemedicine on communication and information transfer in the patient-surgeon relationship.

WHAT IS TELEMEDICINE?

When telemedicine was originally developed, it was based on the assumption that the one-on-one physician and patient relationship was the central focus. In its initial articulation, telemedicine meant a patient receiving services through an electronic medium other than the telephone.[1] Telemedicine has been defined as "the use of medical information exchanged from one site to another via electronic communications to improve patients' health status," whereas "telehealth" encompasses a broader range of health care at a distance that includes more than clinical services.[2] The telemedicine era was heralded in the 1950s when the National Institute of Mental Health connected 7 state hospitals in 4 states through a closed-circuit telephone system,[3] which was soon followed by videoconferencing, transmission of still images, e-health including patient portals, remote monitoring of vital signs, nursing call centers, and continuing medical education, all considered part of telemedicine and telehealth.[2]

Disclosure: The authors have nothing to disclose.
[a] Office of the Vice President for Academic Affairs and Provost, Medical University of South Carolina, 151-B Rutledge Avenue, Room 335, MSC 962, Charleston, SC 29425, USA; [b] Charleston School of Law, 81 Mary Street, Charleston, SC 29403, USA; [c] Department of Surgery, Institute of Human Values in Health Care, Medical University of South Carolina, 25 Courtenay Drive, Suite 7028, MSC 295, Charleston, SC 29425-2950, USA
* Corresponding author. 25 Courtenay Drive, Suite 7028, MSC 295, Charleston, SC 29425-2950.
E-mail address: sader@musc.edu

Thorac Surg Clin 22 (2012) 531–538
http://dx.doi.org/10.1016/j.thorsurg.2012.07.002

THE INTERNET

By the early 1980s, the Internet was launched and soon was recognized as a powerful tool for interaction.[4] Yet, even the most perceptive and knowledgeable students of telemedicine did not predict the rapidity with which computing power, new technology, and modes of usage would develop, and the rapid adoption of electronic communications by the general public was unforeseen. A process that started modestly with electronic mail has expanded to a constantly evolving variety of electronic devices.[5] The Internet has facilitated connection with people and instant access to troves of information. By October 2010, more than two-thirds of households had high-speed Internet access. In 2012, North American users totaled 273 million or 78.6% of the population.[6]

In the United States, 150 million people (66% of all adults, 81% of those online) search for health information online. Patients would like to ask questions of their physicians when a visit is not necessary (77%) and to fix appointments (71%), refill prescriptions (71%), and receive the results of medical tests (70%).[7]

Internet connection was achieved originally only by computer but has been substantially broadened over the last decade by the availability of smaller mobile devices, such as the iPod, the iPhone, and the iPad, which facilitate communication with people and access to information.

PERSPECTIVES AND PERCEPTIONS
Patients

The Internet is used not only to search for health information but also to share experiences of health and illness in social networks. In addition, Internet users, especially caregivers, women, parents with children living at home, and college graduates seek information about physicians or other health professionals.[8] The most common health-related use of the Internet is to ask a physician new questions or seek a second opinion, and a substantial minority (38%) make decisions about whether to see a doctor.[9]

A study from outpatient clinics in large academic primary care centers found that patients using e-mail were younger, better educated, more affluent, and healthier than those who did not use e-mail; women were much more likely to use e-mail than men. Although e-mail users accessed their accounts at home (82%) or at work (57%) and checked their accounts several times each day, 90% of users had never used e-mail to communicate with their physicians; yet, most users (88%) indicated they would be willing to

use e-mail in this way, believing that such communication could improve relationships with their physicians (57%). Nearly half of those who were willing to e-mail their physicians expressed concerns about the effectiveness and efficiency of such communication.[10]

Patients being informed of routine blood test results prefer notification by telephone call (55%), a return visit (20%), a letter (19%), or e-mail (5%).[11] Nearly 30% of the patients in the study were older than 65 years of age, probably contributing to the low preference for e-mail notification, as younger patients and those with higher levels of education were more likely to find notification by e-mail acceptable.

In a study of a large outpatient population, patients preferred e-mail or online communication to obtain prescription renewals, answers to general medical questions, instructions for self-monitoring (eg, blood pressure monitoring), and routine follow-up for minor medical problems. For discussion of healthy lifestyle choices and for reporting of test results, equal numbers favored e-mail/online versus in-person communication. For discussion of treatment options, however, nearly twice as many preferred in-person dialogue to e-mail/online communication. Most patients were not concerned about the confidentiality or privacy of their medical information.[12]

Consumers appraise electronic access to personal health records (PHRs) positively—younger Internet users (18–24 years of age) more so than older (≥65). Ethnicity is an important variable: Hispanics are more likely than non-Hispanic white users to value electronic access to PHRs. People most likely to track their personal information are men, Hispanics, those with a regular health care provider, and those educated beyond high school.[13]

Another large-scale study of attitudes about the potential of health information technology to improve health care found that a large majority (77%) of patients are aware of electronic medical records (EMRs) and favor their use in doctor's offices as part of the office visit. A similar number believe EMRs are likely to improve medical care, and 59% believe EMRs reduce the cost of health care. About 55% of patients value health information technology highly enough to be willing to pay more to broaden its use. About half (48%) of those surveyed indicated they are very concerned about the privacy of medical records, 68% believe that EMRs are secure, and 64% think that the benefits of EMRs outweigh potential risks to privacy. The idea of electronic prescribing is favored by a large majority (80%), and those most likely to believe that e-prescribing improve medical care are patients aged more than or equal to 65 years of age and blacks.[14]

Physicians

Physicians have a broader and more careful approach to Internet communication than most patients. Most primary care physicians (61%) believe that e-mail is a suitable way to reach them and is good for handling the administrative concerns of patients (60%). A smaller majority (52%) do not object to e-mail from patients. Nevertheless, many physicians have important concerns about security and privacy.[10] Even though much guidance on these issues is available, opinions about it still vary widely.[15,16]

A study of physician attitudes found that they believe electronic communication not only has distinct potential benefits, such as reducing the number of nonurgent telephone calls while increasing patient participation in medical decision making, but also has potential for increasing the physician's workload, for inappropriate use in cases of acute serious illnesses, and for legal liability.[17]

Surgical residents' and fellows' attitudes toward e-mail communication have been studied: messages with a colored background, a difficult-to-read font, no salutation, a header with no recipient name, or no subject line are likely to be perceived negatively and the sender to be perceived as inefficient, unprofessional, and irritating. Recipients of such e-mails are unlikely to respond.[18]

Online Social Networks

Interaction between patients and physicians has increased in online social networks (OSNs), such as Facebook, Twitter, MySpace, Friendster, and LinkedIn. Most physicians, including house officers, participate in OSNs for personal use, few for professional purposes.[19] Practicing physicians are more likely than residents and medical students to interact with patients within OSNs, particularly by visiting the profile of a patient or a patient's family and to receive friend requests from patients or their family members. Responding to such requests, 58% of practicing physicians always denied the request, whereas 42% accepted them on a case-by-case basis.

Most physicians and trainees neither find OSNs an ethically appropriate manner to interact or communicate with patients, nor believe OSNs have the potential for improving patient-physician interaction because communication cannot be safely accomplished without compromising patient confidentiality.[19]

The structure and function of OSNs raise questions about the nature of patient-physician boundaries, leading to recommendations that clinicians who use OSNs for interaction with patients should clearly delineate their professional from their social "digital footprint" and constantly be alert to potential patient interactions and lapses in professional integrity. If physicians feel compelled to share access with patients, then they must closely monitor their privacy status and profile content.[19]

Optimizing Clinicians' Time

Asynchronous electronic communications with patients, such as e-mail and online discussions, can enhance the quality and amount of time a physician can devote to patients. Technology promotes handling a larger volume of information in the same amount of time, thus enhancing patient-physician communication. However, 3 claims on a physician's time must be balanced: time with patients, time on documentation, and time on continuing education.[20] The growing medical sophistication of patients through their use of the Internet is reflected in their desire to communicate with clinicians by way of e-mail and other digital technologies. For the clinician, however, electronic communication usually is not reimbursed by third-party payers. Consumption of a valuable limited resource, time, that is not reimbursable can be detrimental to physicians' optimal professional functioning.[21]

Summary of Perspectives and Perceptions

Research using surveys, interviews, and ethnographic methods shows a consistent pattern of increased use of the Internet by patients and their families, as well as a consistent range of questions and concerns. Patients clearly want more Internet interactions with providers in their quest for general information, prescription renewals, and such administrative matters as scheduling appointments. On the other hand, patients prefer in-person communication for treatment instructions. Despite privacy and accuracy concerns, patients are generally satisfied that their communications and medical records are confidential and accurate. Many studies of physicians' perceptions of electronic communication with patients have documented recognition of benefits as well as a consistent chorus of concerns about confidentiality, increased workload, inappropriate use, unreimbursed use of time, and medicolegal issues.[22–24]

ETHICAL AND LEGAL ISSUES IN TELEMEDICINE

Important legal questions emerged as telemedicine developed. Among these are physician licensure, credentialing and privileging, liability (including medical malpractice), reimbursement, and privacy and confidentiality issues.[25,26] Communication between physicians and patients has changed dramatically in the last 5 decades, but, unfortunately, some legal issues have restrained rather than advanced access to telemedicine. The shortage of clinicians in rural areas makes that underserved population especially affected by barriers to telemedicine are elderly and disabled individuals because of their lack of mobility and other health-related conditions. Telemedicine services in private homes as well as long-term care facilities could provide such patients with high-quality, cost-effective primary and specialty care.[27]

The American Medical Association (AMA) Code of Medical Ethics provides e-mail guidelines for physicians, which include the necessity to establish a patient-physician relationship in person, using e-mail only for supplemental encounters, and informing patients clearly about the inherent limitations of e-mail communication.[28] Additional guidelines also require that physicians responsible for health-related websites ensure content accuracy, timeliness, reliability, and scientific soundness, establish safeguards for minimizing conflicts of interest and commercial biases, and provide high-level security protections and privacy-confidentiality safeguards.[29] Inappropriate uses of e-mail include conveying bad news or abnormal or confusing test results, a new problem that requires a complex and dynamic dialogue, or information about sensitive diagnoses, such as human immunodeficiency virus infection, mental illness, disability, or sexually transmitted diseases.[10]

The Federation of State Medical Boards (FSMB) also has promulgated guidelines for physicians who use the Internet in their practices, which are similar to the AMA guidelines but somewhat more detailed. In addition, they include the need for informed consent to "collect, share, or use personal data" and a requirement for the physician to "provide meaningful opportunities for patients to give feedback about their concerns."[30]

Although electronic technology has improved health care and has the potential for even greater improvements, it has also brought new complexities.

Patient-physician Relationship

As technology has progressed, it has become more difficult to determine when and if a patient-physician relationship has been established. In the most traditional sense, a patient-physician relationship is established when a physician examines a patient, makes a diagnosis or treats a patient, and then bills for those services. Courts have held, although, that there can still be a patient-physician relationship even though there has been no direct contact with the patient,[31] and this mirrors the position taken by the AMA: "A patient-physician relationship exists when a physician serves a patient's medical needs, generally by mutual consent between physician and patient (or surrogate). In some instances the agreement is implied, such as in emergency care or when physicians provide services at the request of the treating physician."[32] In ethical terms, it is clear that a patient-physician relationship can exist, even over long distances, without direct contact.

Legally, however, the traditional one-to-one patient-physician relationship comes into question when health care is provided at remote locations, with involvement of multiple professionals, often asynchronously. Whether or not a patient-physician relationship exists when using digital technology for online consultations and for prescribing medications has been confusing. Several courts have grappled with this problem and at least one jurisdiction has held that a patient-physician relationship has not been established when the physician has never seen or examined a new patient in another state, has merely had the patient complete a medical questionnaire, yet prescribes medications over the Internet.[33] However, in at least one jurisdiction, Hawaii, a patient-physician relationship is established through the use of telecommunication devices when the physician holds a valid medical license in Hawaii.[31]

The question of where the practice of medicine actually takes place when the patient is in one place and health care providers in other locations, including different states, presented an early legal challenge. This issue was not an ethical one; however, laws differ by jurisdiction, but physicians' ethical obligations are, for the most part, independent of location. A general consensus has emerged among state licensing boards that the practice of medicine occurs wherever the patient is located, even if the physician's location were in another state.[34]

Medical Licensure

Licensing issues have become a major obstacle to telemedicine.[35] Although much discussion has focused on how to overcome these obstacles, no consensus as to how physicians can proceed with interstate practice has emerged. When a physician practices in a state electronically without a license issued by the licensing board of that state, he or she could potentially be committing a felony.[36] State law varies in requirements to practice telemedicine, but it is not unreasonable to infer that a physician would have to be licensed in all 50 states to practice telemedicine.[37] Ten state boards issue a special practice license, telemedicine license, or certificate or license to practice medicine across state lines to allow for the practice of telemedicine. Most of the state boards and that of the District of Columbia require that a physician be licensed to practice telemedicine in their jurisdictions. At least one state allows out-of-state physicians to practice telemedicine in the state, but the physician must register with the Board.[38]

Practicing medicine across national boundaries is even more cumbersome. The FSMB continues to work on this issue, recognizing the need for a consensus regarding policy aimed at achieving uniformity in providing health care in the age of telemedicine. The FSMB has encouraged states to develop an easier process to facilitate practicing in multiple states.[35]

Physicians involved with telemedicine have faced dire consequences from both civil and criminal perspectives. A court found a physician to have practiced without a license and had not established a patient-physician relationship when she prescribed medications by Internet to various patients across state lines; the physician lost her license.[39] In a criminal case, the court refused to dismiss a criminal complaint against a group of physicians who prescribed medications through the Internet in multiple jurisdictions where they did not possess valid licenses and no patient-physician relationship had existed.[40] A judgment was subsequently entered against the physicians.[41]

Caring for patients in health care facilities with which the physician has no relationship has been problematic in the past because of stringent credentialing and privileging requirements by the Centers for Medicare and Medicaid Services (CMS). CMS has recently eased the requirements for uncredentialed clinicians to practice telemedicine. Among other changes, any Medicare-participating institution that will provide telemedicine services, referred to as the "distant-site hospital," and the hospital receiving the services, the "originating site hospital," must have a written agreement indicating that the distant-site hospital is responsible for meeting the credentialing requirements pursuant to the statute.[42] Still, the rule requires the distant-site physician to be licensed in the state where the originating site services will be provided.[43]

Legal Liability

As with most changes in the way health care is delivered, one can expect that the law will eventually "catch up," and when it does, it may affect malpractice claims related to telemedicine. To date, most of the legal cases involving physicians who are practicing telemedicine relate to prescribing medications by way of the Internet.[44] One may expect to see traditional malpractice claims become more complex as issues such as jurisdiction, procedure, choice of law, and duty of care are injected into the mix.[25] For example, physicians may face lawsuits for failure to diagnose or treat a specific condition because of flawed telemedicine data or faulty telecommunication.[45]

A serious concern for practitioners is the question of the standard of care to which they will be held when practicing telemedicine: will it be the same standard that applies to in-person consultation or will a different standard be specific to telemedicine?[25] Some scholars have suggested that the telemedicine practitioner should be held to a different standard of care in situations where the traditional medical procedures would be distinct from the telemedicine procedures.[46] Through the legislative process, however, Hawaii has already determined that a physician who practices online is held to a lower standard of care than the physician who provides in-person care.[31]

Some professional organizations have provided guidelines for the telemedicine practitioner. The American Telemedicine Association recommends that the practitioner "shall be guided by professional discipline and national existing clinical practice guidelines when practicing via telehealth, and any modifications to specialty-specific clinical practice standards for the telehealth setting shall ensure that clinical requirements specific to the discipline are maintained."[47] Several surgical organizations have also developed guidelines for the telemedicine practitioner. At least one surgical professional organization has developed guidelines that set out specific definitions and appropriate uses for the telecommunication, including remote performance of patient evaluation and consultation, surgery, clinical management, and education for students and other health care professionals.[48]

If telemedicine becomes the standard of care for providing services to rural and underserved areas in the future, a physician may be found liable for failing to recommend telemedicine if his or her peers would have done so under similar circumstances.[25]

Reimbursement

Reimbursement issues have plagued medical practice increasingly in recent decades. Many physicians have expressed concerns related to time management in communicating with their patients by way of e-mail, viewing it as yet another unreimbursed cost. Reimbursement problems also occur when a physician is asked to evaluate or manage a patient's condition remotely. Although Medicare and some Medicaid and private insurance programs pay for some telemedicine services,[49] payment is not consistent and clearly does not consider telemedicine's improvements in access, cost efficiency, and quality of care.

The Patient Protection and Affordable Care Act is designed to take into account innovative ways to deliver quality health care in a cost-effective manner. In fact, the federal government is exploring telemedicine as one of the innovative ways to accomplish this goal.[35]

Informed Consent

The amount of information required to ensure that a patient's consent is adequately informed increases dramatically in telemedicine. Patients may have a great deal of knowledge about their medical conditions and upcoming surgical procedures searching the Internet, but this does not mean that the physician therefore provide less information, rather, more information may be required to correct misinformation the patient has found on the Internet and to explain risks related specifically to telemedicine.

There are 2 questions concerning informed consent: Who is responsible for obtaining the informed consent? (2) What should the patient be told?[25] State law may define who is responsible for obtaining informed consent, but typically, it will be the "distant-site" physician if he or she is talking to the patient directly or is performing a procedure from a remote area.[25] What patients should be told about telemedicine procedures, for example, the possibility that a cardiac monitor may transmit the wrong data, is still evolving.[25] However, informing the patient about all of the known risks and benefits of the technology would be the safer course.[45]

Privacy and Confidentiality Issues

Confidentiality is fundamental to the patient-physician relationship. Unlike the traditional practice of medicine, in which others beside the physician necessarily have access to the patient's information, telemedicine requires even more individuals to have such access, such as the staff responsible for managing the teletechnology. In addition, storage and transmission of the electronic information may be of concern to both physicians and patients. Moreover, patients may not fully appreciate who may be in the room at the distant-site facility during the consult with the specialist.[45] Not obtaining consent that is informed by privacy and confidentiality issues may have dire consequences on many levels, including the patient's dignity and autonomy and the overall well-being of the patient and of the patient-physician relationship.[27]

SUMMARY

The role of telemedicine in the care of patients has been growing steadily for several decades at an accelerating rate over the last 20 years. Its role will continue to expand into the foreseeable future as current benefits are more fully appreciated, potential benefits realized, and existing barriers to its use lowered or eliminated. The greatest value of telemedicine is likely to accrue to underserved populations, patients in rural areas and elderly and disabled persons, but all can benefit from telemedicine technologies in simple ways, such as advice from personal physicians by e-mail or through websites, and to satisfy more demanding needs, such as long-distance consultation with expert specialists.

The scope of this discussion has been limited to the use of digital technologies in communication and information, but telemedicine is broader, including provision of physical services, such as surgery-at-a-distance by robotic technology, which, for example, could allow a surgeon in the United States to repair a dysfunctional mitral valve in a patient lying on an operating table in Europe. Many future uses of electronic technologies in medical practice are unimaginable, just as live television broadcast from a space vehicle to living rooms on Earth, from Apollo 11 in 1969, was literally inconceivable to one of literature's most imaginative and far-seeing novelists, Jules Verne, when he wrote *From the Earth to the Moon* in 1865. The only certainty is that telemedicine is here to stay and has enormous but mostly unrealized potential for enriching the patient-physician relationship.

ACKNOWLEDGMENTS

Dr Sade's role in this publication was supported by the South Carolina Clinical & Translational Research Institute, Medical University of South Carolina's Clinical and Translational Science Award Number UL1RR029882. The contents are solely the responsibility of the authors and do not necessarily represent the official views of the National Center for Research Resources or the National Institutes of Health.

REFERENCES

1. Anika D, Clifton AD. Licensure, reimbursement and liability in telemedicine: an academic perspective. Ann Health Law Advance Directive 2008;18:62–5.

2. American Telemedicine Association. Telemedicine defined. Available at: http://www.americantelemed. org/i4a/pages/index.cfm?pageid=3333. Accessed April 12, 2012.

3. LeVert D. Telemedicine: revamping quality health care in rural America. Ann Health Law Advance Directive 2010;19:215–24.

4. Clark DD. Introduction. Daedalus 2011;140(4):6–14.

5. Horrigan JB. Being disconnected in a broadband-connected world. Daedalus 2011;140(4):19–28.

6. Internet usage statistics. The Internet Big Picture. Internet World Stats: Usage and Population Statistics. Available at: http://www.internetworldstats. com/stats.htm. Accessed April 10, 2012.

7. Patient-physician communication. Harris Interactive Health Care News 2002;2(8):1–4. Available at: http://www.harrisinteractive.com/news/newsletters/ healthnews/HI_HealthCareNews2002Vol2_Iss08.pdf. Accessed April 12, 2002.

8. Fox S. Health topics. Pew Internet. Available at: http://pewInternet.org/Reports/2011/HealthTopics. aspx. Accessed April 12, 2012.

9. Rainie L. The rise of the e-patient: understanding social networks and online health information seeking. Grand Rounds Lecture. Burbank (CA): Providence St. Joseph Medical Center; 2012. Available at: http://www.slideshare.net/PewInternet/ online-health-seeking. Accessed April 12, 2012.

10. Moyer CA, Stern DT, Dobias KS, et al. Bridging the electronic divide: patient and provider perspectives on e-mail communication in primary care. Am J Manag Care 2002;8(5):427–33.

11. Leekha S, Thomas KG, Chaudry R, et al. Patient preferences for and satisfaction with methods of communicating test results in a primary care practice. Joint Comm J Qual Patient Saf 2009;35(10): 497–501.

12. Hassol A, Walker JM, Kidder D, et al. Patient experiences and attitudes about access to a patient electronic health care record and linked web messaging. J Am Med Inform Assoc 2004;11(6):505–13.

13. Wen KY, Kreps G, Zhu F, et al. Consumers' perceptions about and use of the internet for personal health records and health information exchange: analysis of the 2007 health information national trends survey. J Med Internet Res 2010;12(4):e73. Available at: http://www.jmir.org/2010/4/e73. Accessed April 12, 2012.

14. Gaylin DS, Moiduddin A, Mohamoud S, et al. Public attitudes about health information technology, and its relationship to health care quality, costs, and privacy. Health Serv Res 2011;46(3):920–38.

15. Williams SP. Legal aspects of electronic communication. SCMA; 2012. Available at: https://www. scmedical.org/uploads/files/Williams.pdf. Accessed April 12, 2012.

16. Sands DZ. Electronic patient-centered communication: e-mail and other e-ways to communicate clinically. In: Lewis DA, editor. Consumer health informatics: informing consumers and improving health care. New York: Springer; 2005. p. 107–21.

17. Leong SL, Gingrich D, Lewis PR, et al. Enhancing doctor-patient communication using e-mail: a pilot study. J Am Board Fam Pract 2005;18(3):180–8.

18. Resendes S, Ramanan T, Park A, et al. SEND IT: Study of e-mail etiquette and notions from doctors in training. J Surg Educ 2012;69(3):393–403.

19. Bosselt GT, Torke AM, Hickman SE, et al. The patient-doctor relationship and online social networks: results of a national survey. J Gen Intern Med 2011;26(10):1168–74.

20. Wang CJ, Huang AT. Integrating technology into health care: what will it take? JAMA 2012;307(6): 569–70.

21. Herrick DM. Convenient care and telemedicine. NCPA Policy Report No. 305. National Center for Policy Analysis; 2007. Available at:. www.ncpa.org/ pdfs/st305.pdf. Accessed April 12, 2012.

22. Kleiner KD, Akers R, Burke BL, et al. Parent and physician attitudes regarding electronic communication in pediatric practices. Pediatrics 2002; 109(5):740–4.

23. Ventres W, Kooienga S, Vuckovic N, et al. Physicians, patients and the electronic health record: an ethnographic analysis. Ann Fam Med 2006;4(2): 124–31.

24. Ferguson T. Digital doctoring—opportunities and challenges in electronic patient-physician communication. JAMA 1998;280(15):1361–2.

25. Hoffman D, Rowthorn V. Legal impediments to the diffusion of telemedicine. J Health Care Law Pol 2011;14:1–53.

26. Carnell H. How Illinois is using telemedicine to improve health care access in rural communities. Public Interest Law Reporter 2008;13:159–67.

27. Fleming D, Edison K, Pak H. Telehealth ethics. Telemed J E Health 2009;15(8):797–803.

28. Council on Ethical and Judicial Affairs. Opinion 5.026, the use of electronic mail. In: AMA, editor. Code of medical ethics: current opinions with annotations. 2010-2011th edition. Chicago: American Medical Association; 2010. p. 153–5.

29. Council on Ethical and Judicial Affairs. Opinion 5.027, use of health-related online sites. In: AMA, editor. Code of medical ethics: current opinions with annotations. 2010-2011th edition. Chicago: American Medical Association; 2010. p. 155–6.

30. Federation of State Medical Boards of the United States. FSMB model guidelines for appropriate use

of internet in the medical practice. Available at: http://www.fsmb.org/pdf/2002_grpol_Use_of_Internet.pdf. Accessed April 12, 2012.

31. Bailey R. The legal, financial, and ethical implications of online medical consultations. Journal of Technology Law and Policy 2011;16:53–105.

32. Council on Ethical and Judicial Affairs. Opinion 10.015, The Patient-physician relationship. In: AMA, editor. Code of medical ethics: current opinions with annotations. 2010-2011th edition. Chicago: American Medical Association; 2010. p. 374–7.

33. Golob v Arizona Medical Board, 217 Ariz 505, 509 (2008).

34. Ameringer CF. State-based licensure of telemedicine: the need for uniformity but not a national scheme. J Health Care Law Pol 2011;14:55–85.

35. Federation of State Medical Boards. Balancing access, safety, and quality in a new era of telemedicine, summary and highlights, a conference to discuss telemedicine's future. Washington, DC. 2011. p. 9. Available at: www.fsmb.org/pdf/pub-symposium-telemed.pdf. Accessed April 12, 2012.

36. Federation of State Medical Boards. Essentials of modern medical and osteopathic practice act. 12th edition. 2010. p. 26. Available at: http://www.fsmb.org/pdf/GRPOL_essentials.pdf. Accessed April 12, 2012.

37. Siegal G. Enabling globalization of health care in the information technology era: telemedicine and the medical world wide web. Va J Law Tech 2012;17:1–34.

38. Federation of State Medical Boards of the United States. Telemedicine overview board by board approach. Available at: http://www.fsmb.org/pdf/GRPOL_Telemedicine_Licensure.pdf. Accessed April 12, 2012.

39. Golob v Arizona Medical Board of State, 217 Ariz 505 (2008).

40. U.S. v Rodriguez, 532 F Supp 2d 316 (D.P.R. 2007).

41. U.S. Motion to Unseal Judgments, U.S. v Rodriguez, No. 07–032 (JAG) (D.P.R. May 4, 2010), ECF No. 620.

42. 42 C.F.R. § 482.12(a)(1)-(a)(9) (2011) for hospitals; 42C.F.R. § 485.616 (c) (1) (i-vii) (2011) for critical access hospitals (CAH).

43. Melnik T, Balow B. Revisions to telemedicine credentialing and privileging rules. J Health Care Compl 2011;13(4):41–4.

44. Golob, 217 Ariz 505 (2008); Rodriguez, 532 F Suppp 2d 316 (D.P.R. 2007).

45. Kupchynsky R, Camin C. Legal considerations of telemedicine. Texas Bar J 2001;64:20–8.

46. Rannefeld L. The doctor will e-mail you now: physician's use of telemedicine to treat patients over the Internet. J Law Health 2004;19:75–105.

47. American Telemedicine Association. Core standards for telemedicine operations, clinical standards. 2007. Available at: http://www.americantelemed.org/files/public/standards/CoreStandards_withCOVER.pdf. Accessed April 12, 2012.

48. Society of American Gastrointestinal and Endoscopic Surgeons. Guidelines for the surgical practice of telemedicine. Available at: http://www.sages.org/publication/id/21/. Accessed April 12, 2012.

49. Bennett J. Improving quality of care through telemedicine: the need to remove reimbursement and licensure barriers. Annals of Health Law Advance Directive 2010;19:203–14.

Patients' Perspective in the Surgical Decision-Making Process

Eric Lim, MB ChB, MD, MSc (Biostatistics), FRCS (C-Th)

KEYWORDS

- Patient preferences • Decision making • Surgical management • Information

KEY POINTS

- Barriers can arise if surgeons are unable to effectively convey information on benefits and risks or are unwilling to offer management choices based on patients' preferences.
- Facilitating shared decision making, allowing patients to carefully think and consider the alternatives, and empowering them to share in the decision-making process improve patient satisfaction and treatment adherence and represent the hallmark of an excellent clinician.

INTRODUCTION

There are 2 types of clinicians who allow patients to decide their management plan: the worst of doctors and the best of doctors. The paradox is easily explained. The first is the uninformed doctor, who is unaware of the available options and corresponding benefits and risks and therefore relies on the patient to decide what he or she thinks is preferable. The second is the fully informed doctor with a thorough knowledge and grounding of the subject who is able to detail the management options and corresponding benefits and risks and has the confidence to inform the patient when he or she does not know the answer (because there is no available evidence) to guide the decision and helps the patient decide the best management option. Most clinicians tend to practice safely in the middle by following recommendations (of others) published in textbooks or, more often, national or international guidelines (written by others) that are designed for the population as a whole rather than the person who is sitting on the other side of the clinician's desk.

Unfortunately, patient perception in the surgical decision-making process is not a well-researched field in thoracic surgery, and much of what is written in this article is based on the author's experience quantifying benefits and risks on a wide range of medical and surgical procedures as an editor of a textbook of medicine and surgery,[1] understanding clinical decision making at empiric levels as a qualified medical statistician, awareness of the difficulties in appreciation and communication of benefits and risk as a final-year undergraduate teacher at Imperial College Medical School in London, and aware, as a practicing surgeon, of the difficulties patients face when attempting to come to terms with major life-changing decisions.

SURGICAL DECISION MAKING

At the most basic level, surgical decision making seems simple: the benefits and risks of each procedure are weighed and a decision undertaken in favor of the option whereby the benefit outweighs the risk. The difficulties arise in this decision, however, when trying to establish the size of the benefit against the size of the risk. To take things one step further, it is not simply the benefit or risk as quantified by a number (eg, a 28% risk of a recurrence of a spontaneous pneumothorax

The Academic Division of Thoracic Surgery, The Royal Brompton Hospital, Sydney Street, London SW3 6NP, UK
E-mail address: e.lim@rbht.nhs.uk

Thorac Surg Clin 22 (2012) 539–543
http://dx.doi.org/10.1016/j.thorsurg.2012.07.001
1547-4127/12/$ – see front matter © 2012 Elsevier Inc. All rights reserved.

after the first episode[2]) but the *perceived* risk (eg, whether is 28% an important or unimportant threshold for the recurrence of a pneumothorax). Perceived risk is much more difficult, if not impossible, to interpret. In the pneumothorax example, a 28% recurrence risk may be a very different number when interpreted by a young man aspiring to be an accountant who developed a small pneumothorax treated by observation only versus a young man aspiring to be a deep sea diver who developed a tension pneumothorax and had extensive difficulties getting access to medical treatment. Older "guidelines" for the management of pneumothorax tended to recommend surgery only after the second episode,[3] whereas more recently, the influence of patient choice is taken into consideration for surgery after the first episode.[4]

Doctors Know Best?

In 2008, the General Medical Council of the United Kingdom issued recommendations on obtaining consent for procedures, encouraging doctors to share the decision-making process with patients.[5] The General Medical Council recommended that the benefits and risks are conveyed to patients, who are allowed to decide on the best course of action. Most important, the guidance document recommended that the decision may be undertaken by the patient for reasons that the doctor does not agree with or for no reason at all. The guidance places the patient firmly in the "driving seat" with regard to the course of clinical management, and this does not always sit well with clinicians who have a strong paternal approach to patient management. Ultimately, whether it is an international guideline or individual clinician, our recommendations are shaped by our collective (guidelines committees) or personal *subjective* interpretation of benefits and risk. This only works well if this is in-line with the patients' subjective interpretations, and the remaining sections underscore the importance of establishing the patient's standpoint.

The "Best" Option

Clinicians often think that patients always want the best option. This is far from the truth. The author conducted a systematic review and meta-analysis of the risk of recurrence after surgery for pneumothorax and concluded that access is one of the most important influencing factors for recurrence, with open pleurectomy having the lowest risk of recurrence (1%) and thoracoscopic pleurectomy having a risk of recurrence of 4%.[6] Because it is relatively straightforward to perform the procedure open or thoracoscopically, patients in my practice were given a choice of access and, to my surprise, approximately two-thirds choose a thoracoscopic procedure with the antecedent higher recurrence risk. The reasons for choosing a thoracoscopic approach are usually the perceptions of less pain and better cosmetic result. In this subset of patients, an absolute difference of 3% in the 2 approaches is unimportant. On the other hand, the minority of patients who chose an open approach often cite the importance of having the best possible outcome, and in their minds, the 4-fold reduction in the risk of recurrence with open surgery is important. This example nicely illustrates the points that the interpretation of a 3% risk difference is different from patient to patient (and certainly with guideline committees[4]), and the difficulty in recommending the "best" option is that the outcome of importance may be different between doctors, who are focused on recurrence rates, and patients, who consider to be pain and cosmesis equally (if not more) important.

Benefits and Risks: The Lung Cancer Paradox

In numerous cases, it is possible to quantify a benefit for a procedure. For example, after the first episode of a pneumothorax, the untreated risk of recurrence is 28%,[2] reducing to 1% if an open pleurectomy is undertaken.[6] The risks of surgery are usually well documented and can be obtained by a retrospective review of the practice of each surgeon.

Sometimes the benefits of a proposed treatment or management option cannot be quantified. The most pertinent example is surgery for early-stage lung cancer. There has never been a study comparing surgery for early-stage lung cancer to an untreated control group[7] and, therefore, in this respect, the benefits on survival cannot be quantified. Some consider that surgery is the only form of "cure," but the use of "cure" in this setting is questionable because after surgery the most important determinant of survival is pathologic stage. If surgery was genuinely "curative," there would only be one survival plot for all stages (because all resected disease has been removed whether a patient is in stage IA or IIB, the survival should be identical). Even at the most optimistic estimates, the survival of patients with stage IA disease does not approach that of the age- and sex-matched population without cancer. Many would consider a randomized trial to be unethical; however, the question remains important in clinical practice. As age and comorbidities increase, so do surgical mortality and morbidity. Although it seems easy for the young, fit patients with early-stage lung cancer to make a decision in favor of surgical resection, where does that leave the older patients with multiple comorbidities and, more important, all those patients who are between these 2 extremes? This question is especially difficult for clinicians to evaluate because the 2 arms of the equation are unbalanced—clinicians can quantify risk (eg, using a logistic model such as Thoracoscore[8]) but cannot quantify the benefit (vs no surgical treatment). In this setting of clinical uncertainty, patients' views and perceptions that influence the decision going forward are critical.

Dealing with Uncertainty

The best doctors pride themselves in being able to make a management decision based on clear risk-benefit analysis, but, as described in the earlier lung cancer example, it is not always possible to quantify or express the benefit to the patient. In the presence of such uncertainty, there are 2 approaches. The easiest is for the surgeon to emphasize his or her expertise and formulate an opinion based on his or her values; the more difficult approach is to admit that the surgeon is unable to quantify the benefit and allow the patient to decide on the best course of management based on individual preference.

Another common scenario in which uncertainty occurs is when there is no clear evidence of a difference in benefit between 2 management options, such as the optimum management of patients with clinical N2 disease. There has never been more evidence generated on this topic in the history of surgery for lung cancer, yet it results in the most uncertainty in clinical practice. This is because the 5 randomized trials to date have not shown any difference between the overall survival of patients with clinical N2 disease who received induction treatment (chemotherapy or chemoradiotherapy) and were randomly assigned to surgery or to radiotherapy.[9–13] Clinicians and guideline committee members often struggle when it comes to equipoise in the evidence. Proponents of medical treatment argue that medical therapy is not as invasive as surgery and should be considered the "standard of care," but there is no difference in the "benefit" of overall survival and therefore the decision rests on the perceptions of acceptability of the risks between the 2, and of the patient's preference of the treatment modality. The "evidence" supports the patient's choice for surgery if the patient is more comfortable with the idea of complete surgical resection and systematic nodal dissection as a shorter form of treatment. British Guidelines on the Radical Management of Patients with Lung

Cancer allowed leeway in the recommendations to present the perceived benefits and risks for patients to decide in this setting.[14]

Moving the argument forward, even if the patient's perspective in surgical decision making is embraced, potential barriers with the surgeon, patient, or doctor–patient interaction may still prevent joint decision making.

ROLE OF THE SURGEON
Understanding and Conveying Information on Risk

If surgeons subscribe to the notion that patients should be allowed to make their own independent decision regarding benefits and risks, he or she still needs to quantify it to facilitate the correct interpretation. An intermediate understanding of statistics is usually required, a subject often poorly taught in medical school and not usually covered in surgical training. The most basic level is the ability to convey percentage risk. For example, the risk of in-hospital death after lobectomy is approximately 3%[15]; this does not mean that the chance of death is 3% but that, on average, in cohorts of 100 patients (exactly like yourself), 3 of every 100 with die in hospital as a direct result of lobectomy.

As quantification of benefit becomes more sophisticated in the literature (eg, whereby benefits are expressed as a hazard ratio), clinicians would need to have a greater level of understanding of statistics. The author and colleagues surveyed British surgeons, physicians, and oncologists regarding whether they were able to calculate the expected benefits of adjuvant chemotherapy based on the published benefit stated as a hazard ratio of 0.80. The results suggested that 33% of surgeons, 53% of physicians, and 73% of oncologists were able to correctly calculate the expected survival of patients.[16] Although such a standard of proficiency in statistics cannot be expected of all doctors, one cannot quantify the benefit to patients if he or she is unable to express the benefit in simple terms, such as a proportion, that the patient can understand. If this were to be the case, then either the surgeon would need to seek help with the definition of "benefit" (Web site, tables) or defer the discussion and allow the patient to have the discussion with someone else who would be able to confer the expected benefits in lay terms. Our results suggested that oncologists were expected to be the group best able to undertake this task.

Flexibility in Surgical Approach

Other examples of flexibility in practice include offering patients a range of procedures based on their preferences. With experience in clinical practice, surgeons tend to have a preference for management, such as the extent of lung resection for cancer. Recommendations for either anatomic lobectomy or wedge resection are based on perceived assessment of lung function and risk rather than on a discussion with the patient. This is not a problem in most patients, who have good lung function and to whom anatomic resection, the procedure with the lower recurrence rate,[17] is offered. Patient opinion becomes increasingly important in the presence of poor lung function, when patients may decide on anatomic lung resection if their concerns about cancer recurrence are higher than that of postoperative shortness of breath, and vice versa. The most evident gesture of respecting patient choice is for the surgeon to refer on to another colleague if the patient would like a procedure or access that is not offered.

ROLE OF THE PATIENT
Patient Expectations

Although much of this article has focused on the decision-making process and on doctors facilitating such an approach, occasionally, patients do not want to engage in a decision-making process. This is usually based on expectations that the patient is seeking a medical consultation and wants the doctor to make a recommendation, and clearly the simplest and easiest way is to comply. One wonders, however, if it is the best or correct way, because patients often assume that decisions are made at a complex and esoteric level. In most of the time, this is not the case. The decision for the patient accepting the risk of surgery is a good example, and patients may expect the doctor to make a recommendation (either for or against surgery). Surgeons are unable to frame the benefits based on improved survival in early-stage lung cancer compared with medical treatment, as explained in the section on cancer "paradox," and therefore tend to frame it as acceptable risk. Surgeons assume that the benefits of surgery in patients with a low risk of death and complications would outweigh the risk. However, clinicians also tend to assume that the level and risk threshold of the patient are the same as for the clinican (eg, 2% risk of death is low and 20% is very high), but this is clearly not the case. The author has met several patients in whom a risk of death of 2% for lung resection has been considered unacceptably high, and when delivering a lecture on the risk for surgery to patients, the author often surveys the audience to determine where "acceptable" risk lies, being

surprised to see hands still raised indicating acceptable risk at levels as high as 50%!

Level of Understanding

Clearly one evident barrier is the level of understanding of the patient. Not all patients are able to comprehend proportions sufficiently well to be able to actively participate in surgical decision making, a problem that can be effectively addressed in many cases by a simple quantification of "high," "low," or "serious" level of risk.

Unable to Make a Choice

Rarely, patients understand the risks involved but simply cannot decide on the best option, and this is often best addressed by breaking down the individual components (eg, concerns about the cancer spreading if untreated against the concerns of the risk of death during surgery) to clarify the thought process in helping patients to decide.

The Right Choice?

Perhaps one of the most important questions to consider is whether patients are satisfied with the decisions that they have made. The author and colleagues have conducted a retrospective study in patients with poor lung function with a predicted postoperative forced expiratory volume in 1 second or carbon monoxide transfer factor less than 40% who were referred for surgery, to determine in those who chose surgical treatment versus those who choice medical therapy whether the patients were satisfied with their choise.[18] When given the opportunity to consider the options and participate in the surgical decision, patients tend to make the correct choices for themselves. This has been substantiated in systematic reviews of shared decision making regarding patient satisfaction and treatment adherence.[19]

SUMMARY

At the most basic level, surgical decision making involves an assessment of benefits against risk. However, in practice, it may not always be possible to quantify benefits; patients may not have the same perception of value or risk and, in many cases, there is uncertainty or equipoise. In this setting, patients' perceptions are critical to the management decision. Barriers can arise if surgeons are unable to effectively convey information on benefits and risks or are unwilling to offer management choices based on patients' preferences. In addition, not all patients expect or want to be involved in the decision-making process; some are unable to clearly understand the benefits or risks and some are genuinely unable to decide. Doctor–patient communication can be achieved by breaking down barriers. Presenting benefits and risks in a simple manner and deconstructing the decision process into components that are perceived to be important to the patient help overcome some of these barriers. Facilitating shared decision making, allowing patients to carefully think and consider the alternatives, and empowering them to share in the decision improves patient satisfaction and treatment adherence and is the hallmark of an excellent clinician.

REFERENCES

1. Lim E, Loke YK, Thompson A. Medicine and surgery: an integrated textbook. Edinburgh (United Kingdom): Elsevier; 2007.

2. Baumann MH, Strange C. Treatment of spontaneous pneumothorax: a more aggressive approach? Chest 1997;112(3):789–804.

3. Baumann MH, Strange C, Heffner JE, et al. Management of spontaneous pneumothorax: an American College of Chest Physicians Delphi consensus statement. Chest 2001;119(2):590–602.

4. MacDuff A, Arnold A, Harvey J. Management of spontaneous pneumothorax: British Thoracic Society Pleural Disease Guideline 2010. Thorax 2010;65(Suppl 2):ii18–31.

5. General Medical Council. Consent: patients and doctors making decisions together. London: General Medical Council; 2008.

6. Barker A, Maratos EC, Edmonds L, et al. Recurrence rates of video-assisted thoracoscopic versus open surgery in the prevention of recurrent pneumothoraces: a systematic review of randomised and non-randomised trials. Lancet 2007;370(9584):329–35.

7. Wright G, Manser RL, Byrnes G, et al. Surgery for non-small cell lung cancer: systematic review and meta-analysis of randomised controlled trials. Thorax 2006;61(7):597–603.

8. Falcoz PE, Conti M, Brouchet L, et al. The Thoracic Surgery Scoring System (Thoracoscore): risk model for in-hospital death in 15,183 patients requiring thoracic surgery. J Thorac Cardiovasc Surg 2007; 133(2):325–32.

9. Johnstone DW, Byhardt RW, Ettinger D, et al. Phase III study comparing chemotherapy and radiotherapy with preoperative chemotherapy and surgical resection in patients with non-small-cell lung cancer with spread to mediastinal lymph nodes (N2); final report of RTOG 89–01. Radiation Therapy Oncology Group. Int J Radiat Oncol Biol Phys 2002;54(2):365–9.

10. Shepherd FA, Johnston MR, Payne D, et al. Randomized study of chemotherapy and surgery versus radiotherapy for stage IIIA non-small-cell lung cancer: a National Cancer Institute of Canada Clinical Trials Group Study. Br J Cancer 1998; 78(5):683–5.

11. Stephens RJ, Girling DJ, Hopwood P, et al. A randomised controlled trial of pre-operative chemotherapy followed, if feasible, by resection versus radiotherapy in patients with inoperable stage T3, N1, M0 or T1-3, N2, M0 non-small cell lung cancer. Lung Cancer 2005;49(3):395–400.

12. van Meerbeeck JP, Kramer GW, Van Schil PE, et al. Randomized controlled trial of resection versus radiotherapy after induction chemotherapy in stage IIIA-N2 non-small-cell lung cancer. J Natl Cancer Inst 2007;99:442–50.

13. Albain KS, Swann RS, Rusch VW, et al. Radiotherapy plus chemotherapy with or without surgical resection for stage III non-small-cell lung cancer: a phase III randomised controlled trial. Lancet 2009;374(9687):379–86.

14. Lim E, Baldwin D, Beckles M, et al. Guidelines on the radical management of patients with lung cancer. Thorax 2010;65(Suppl 3):iii1–27.

15. Page R, Keogh B. National thoracic surgery activity and outcomes report. Oxford (United Kingdom): Dendrite Clinical Systems Ltd; 2008.

16. Khor KS, Tai D, Popat S, et al. Oncologists', physicians' and surgeons' opinions on the perceived value and appropriateness of the specialty to inform patients on adjuvant chemotherapy after radical surgery for non-small cell lung cancer. J Clin Oncol 2011;29(Suppl) [abstract: 7011].

17. Ginsberg RJ, Rubinstein LV. Randomized trial of lobectomy versus limited resection for T1 N0 non-small cell lung cancer. Lung Cancer Study Group. Ann Thorac Surg 1995;60(3):615–22 [discussion: 622–3].

18. Pattenden H, Karunanantham J, Leung M, et al. Functional outcome in patients with non-small cell lung cancer who failed BTS recommended post-operative predicted criteria for lung resection. Lung Cancer 2010;67:S37.

19. Joosten EA, DeFuentes-Merillas L, de Weert GH, et al. Systematic review of the effects of shared decision-making on patient satisfaction, treatment adherence and health status. Psychother Psychosom 2008;77(4):219–26.

Patient Safety in the Surgical Setting

M. Blair Marshall, MD*, Dominic Emerson, MD

KEYWORDS

- Patient safety • Surgical risk • Complications • Morbidity • Mortality • Communication

KEY POINTS

- Constant vigilance is needed to protect patients from error.
- Surgeons work in an increasingly hazardous environment defined by the complexity of care, further specialization, a more challenging patient population, and increased hand-offs among providers.
- Surgeons need to embrace the cultural change necessary to study errors prospectively, learn from their occurrence, and continually implement change to prevent future occurrences.
- Surgeons need to be strong advocates for this continual change within the system to help the surgical team trap errors before they reach the patients.
- Only through a conscious, robust team approach to error identification and management can surgeons slowly move toward safer health care for all.

INTRODUCTION

The publications on a subject can be a telling sign of the level of interest in that subject; a PubMed search for "patient safety" within 2011 yields more than 1900 results, whereas the same search yields 27 documents in 1990. Much of the current public and government-directed attention to patient safety within the United States stems from the 1999 Institute of Medicine report *To Err Is Human*, which estimated that nearly 100,000 deaths annually are the result of medical errors.[1] While the Institute of Medicine report was groundbreaking in its breadth and public nature of its presentation, surgeons have been addressing patient safety and outcomes for almost 100 years.

Many of the advances seen today with regard to patient safety began with attempts to improve outcomes within the surgical population. During the early 1900s in the United States, Dr Ernest Codeman of the Massachusetts General Hospital set out to examine patient outcomes within the surgical population with a goal of improving patient care.

From this research, he came to the conclusion that standardization of care based on current evidence was essential to advancing medicine into the new century. This early work attracted the attention of a fledgling society, the American College of Surgeons, and in the year of its official founding, the college appointed Dr Codeman to chair a committee on hospital standardization. From this appointment he would go on to create the American College of Surgeons Hospital Standardization Program, which would eventually grow separate from the college and become the Joint Commission on Accreditation of Healthcare Organizations and then The Joint Commission. Today, this is the largest health care accreditation body in the United States.

It is estimated that 40% to 50% of hospital errors take place in the operating room.[1,2] Errors contribute to the development of complications in more than half of reported complications, and the rate may be even higher.[3] Errors occurring in the surgical setting are often as complex as the environments in which they occur. Although the review of errors that result in harm often focus on

Division of Thoracic Surgery, Department of Surgery, Georgetown University Medical Center, 3800 Reservoir Rd NW, Washington, DC 20007, USA
* Corresponding author.
E-mail address: MBM5@gunet.georgetown.edu

Thorac Surg Clin 22 (2012) 545–550
http://dx.doi.org/10.1016/j.thorsurg.2012.07.004
1547-4127/12/$ – see front matter © 2012 Elsevier Inc. All rights reserved.

the "sharp end," human error, the actual occurrence of errors is more complex than that. Factors related to the specific systems, processes, and personnel all contribute to the occurrence from error, but systems issues are involved in 90% of errors resulting in adverse events.

The surgical setting represents a complex set of events among several teams, including multiple "hand-offs" to complete care. This coordination represents a highly complex set of events where the opportunity for errors at any point in time is significant and further compounded by the intensity of events. Although the numbers of events that occur in the entire surgical setting have never been defined as a denominator, in a prospective study of intensive care, errors occurred only 1% of the time, but this averaged out to 1.7 events per patient per day.[4]

In the late 1980s and early 1990s, the Society of Anesthesiology used the analysis of closed claims data to identify areas for improvement.[5] The initial project, an analysis of 14 patients who sustained cardiac arrest during spinal anesthesia, resulted in the routine use of pulse oximetry and epinephrine resuscitation. These and many more important findings from the analysis of rare devastating events led to the marked improvement in the safety of anesthesia with the now routine use of pulse oximetry, capnography, and other standard devices.[6] Other groups have attempted to use closed claims data to identify similar patterns of errors; however, the impact of these studies has not yet reached the same level.

There is much to be learned from error identification and management in other high-risk industries.[7,8] The groundwork on error identification and management came from similar work done in the aviation industry. James Reason's work highlights the process of errors and how they occur, and this has been adapted to surgery. Errors often occur as the result of a cumulative act effect, a combination of latent and active failures that eventually results in an event that causes harm to the patient (**Fig. 1**).

Human error is inevitable. As long as humans are involved in the care of the patient, errors will occur. However, an intricate knowledge of the system within which one works and the latent errors that exist will help to mitigate errors and, it is hoped, prevent them from reaching the patient. It is a rare event when an error reaches a patient; a more common scenario is when it is trapped or mitigated, the "near miss" event. Near miss events occur 4 to 20 times more frequently than do actual adverse events, and much of this variance depends on the retrospective or prospective nature of the study. Given the propensity for error and the magnitude

of adverse events, such as wrong-site surgery, the analysis of errors had led to significant improvements in the systems-based approach. Identification and prevention of errors occurs through a multitude of mechanisms, and the authors have outlined some tools available for analysis and prevention.

ANALYSIS OF ERRORS
Identification of Errors

Traditionally, surgeons have historically reported and peer reviewed outcomes in the form of morbidity and mortality reports. This typically represents a "blame" type of culture, placing the responsibility solely on the shoulders of the surgeon. Although results have improved as the complexity of procedures has continued to rise, this is not sufficient where the occurrence of error is concerned.[9] Errors associated with complications analyzed in this fashion are rarely captured as such and prevent the systems-based analysis required for thorough evaluation. A systems-based approach to reporting and analysis, ideally one that is mandatory, would be more apt to identify the factors contributing the occurrences of errors, specifically the "latent issues" and personnel.

Error-Reporting Systems

Sentinel event reporting
A sentinel event is defined as any unanticipated event that results in death or serious injury to a patient. Although there may be a broad range of errors that fall into this category, The Joint Commission also has a specific list of events, including wrong-site surgery and surgical instrument or object left in a patient, that require reporting and a root-cause analysis. Reporting of these events is mandatory, and part of this process includes creation of an "action plan" aimed at reducing the occurrence of such events in the future.

Adverse event reporting
Not all adverse events qualify as sentinel events, but a similar analysis of events may still lead to the identification of system and other latent errors predisposing to the occurrence of errors. Error reporting is currently performed on institutional, state, or nationwide levels and may be entirely voluntary or mandatory. Voluntary reporting systems are not as effective as mandatory systems but may be all that is available, depending on the institution.[10] Systems-based issues can be addressed and improvements made as a result from the analysis of such events.

Near miss analysis
Not all errors result in harm to the patient; there may be recovery from error, the "trapped errors."

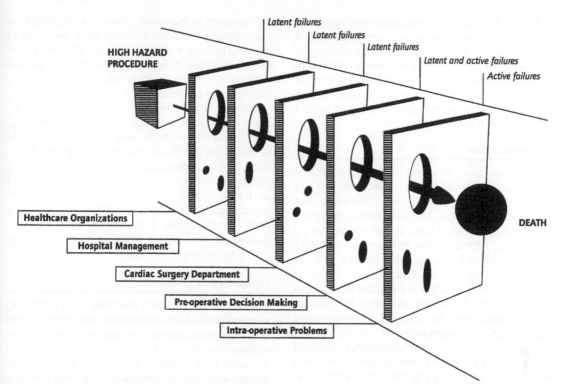

Fig. 1. Organizational model of errors applied to health care. (*From* Carthey J, de Leval MR, Reason JT. The human factor in cardiac surgery: errors and near misses in a high technology medical domain. Ann Thorac Surg 2001;72(1):300–5; with permission, and Reason JT. Human error. Cambridge [United Kingdom]: Cambridge University Press; 1990.)

It is estimated that near miss events are 4 to 20 times more common than events which actually harm the patient. Analysis of these events can lead to the identification of system and personnel issues with improvements made to prevent actual harm from reaching the patients.[11] Also, near miss analysis allows for the identification and acknowledgment of those responsible for recovery from these errors, identifying areas of strength and often effective teamwork within the system.

PREVENTION OF ERROR
Systems Approach

Although human error is the direct cause of many adverse events, other high-reliability organizations have adopted a systems-based approach to mitigate errors. Systems can be contributory or protective in the occurrence of errors, and this concept is critical in the design and implementation of systems in the medical industry. As an example, hospitals may purchase a piece of equipment based on best price instead of the most effective design to prevent errors. The latter, a human factors approach, encourages equipment design for ease of use and error minimization. This type of approach may steer the system

toward error entrapment instead of responding to adverse events. In designing systems to minimize error, as a result of adverse events, it must be recognized that one cannot always predict success. Every intervention to improve safety may reduce errors associated with a previously identified risk but may also create a new unanticipated consequence that may contribute to the development of new errors and the potential for harm. Patient safety is a moving target.

Crew Resource Management

Crew resource management (CRM) has been effectively used by the aviation industry to successfully manage potential errors.[12] The most important aspect of CRM for medical error identification and correction has been the method by which CRM addresses errors. CRM separates error protection into 3 categories: prevention, detection, and recovery—an approach that lends itself well to medicine as a whole, and in particular, surgery. CRM seeks to primarily prevent errors from happening, but also acknowledges that errors will still occur and that they must be quickly identified and remedied within the context of a rapidly changing and high-risk industry. In addition, given the team-oriented care provided in the operating room, including anesthesia and nursing personnel and surgeons, CRM is a natural fit for the complexity of the surgical setting. This systematic evaluation of errors and error sources has improved patient safety as a whole, and from these evaluations many new recommendations for the administration of patient care have been established.

Communication

Communication continues to be a major source of errors and adverse events. Because of the fractionizing of medical care following the implementation of the 80-hour workweek, errors during patient handoff have become increasingly scrutinized. Although the consensus regarding how to deal with this potential source of error is still building, it is obvious that ensuring adequate communication is essential to reducing risk to patients.[13] Recent attempts to improve care handoffs have focused on communication tools, such as computerized records, that facilitate transfer of care.[14] Additional research in the development of formal communication strategies in an attempt to mitigate communication errors has also become prominent.[15] Many groups have begun to incorporate formalized communication handoffs in either a structured, situation-background-assessment-recommendation, or checklist format.[16–18] However, the ideal strategy remains to be seen.

Sterile Cockpit

Along with other lessons learned from aviation safety, the concept of the "sterile cockpit" has been increasing discussed. This relates to the critical high-risk phases of flight, namely takeoff and landing, where nonessential activities are prohibited. Anesthesia clinicians have adopted an analogous parallel—namely, induction and emergence from anesthesia.[19] However, the operating room is a more complex environment than of an airplane. In our setting, the "sterile cockpit" concept is not truly applicable because this period varies for each team. For example, the "sterile cockpit" period for anesthesia is induction and emergence; for surgeons, it is during the critical phases of the operation; and for nurses, it may be when the patient enters the room and when closing occurs, ensuring accurate instrument counts and specimen reconciliation.

Preoperative Marking

Wrong-site surgery is an error that should never occur. Thoracic surgery is particularly at risk, compared with cardiac or general surgery, given the laterality of the chest. Given the magnitude of such an error, several systems have been put in place to prevent such occurrences. Despite layers of preventative measures including formal site verification, surgical "timeouts," and so forth, these errors continue to occur.

Several contributing factors may lead to the initiation of wrong-site surgery: patient positioning, anesthesia interventions, failure to verify consents or markings, and failure to perform a proper timeout. Sources of rescue include patients, circulating nurses, and verifying consents. It is interesting that at times, the formal timeout processes were unsuccessful in preventing "wrong" surgery. This work demonstrates that verification of patient, procedure, and site is required at multiple time points to recover from error.[20]

Preoperative Checklist

Given the morbidity and mortality associated with surgical procedures worldwide, the World Health Organization examined the use of a preoperative surgical checklist and its impact on morbidity and mortality in a global population.[21] They demonstrated improved outcomes following the incorporation of a preoperative surgical checklist. There are several advantages to the use of a checklist. (1) It ensures that the key players in the operating room share the same mental model of anticipated events to occur. (2) It ensures that the needed instrumentation, blood products, etc, are available. (3) It encourages flattening of the hierarchy in surgery and effective teamwork. (4) It ensures that everyone understands the relative risk and anticipated events associated with the procedure. (5) It can also be used to highlight compliance with safety regulations such as timing of preoperative antibiotics and need for a perioperative β-blocker.

Given the outcomes, the Society of Thoracic Surgeon's Workforce on Patient Safety adapted the World Health Organization surgical checklist to one specific for general thoracic procedures. This can be freely downloaded and modified for use by anyone at any institution (www.sts.org/sites/default/files/documents/pdf/ndb/GT_from_Checklists.pdf). The additional impact of such a checklist has been demonstrated through a retrospective analysis of closed malpractice claims. In one study, the authors determined that the use of a preoperative checklist may have prevented 40% of deaths and 29% of permanent injury in the cases they reviewed.[22]

Postoperative Care

In-hospital improvements directed at patient safety have been a popular target by much of the recent work on the subject, and recommendations have been made on several issues, many of which have already been implemented by various regulatory bodies.

As opposed to safety interventions in the operating room, much of the focus of improving in-hospital safety has been aimed at improving the system in which the care is delivered. Many of the current recommendations for improving safety in thoracic surgery are the same for all hospital-based medical teams. One of the most controversial of these, at least in the minds of most surgeons, is the duty hour restriction. It has been found that limiting resident work hours limits errors in some studies,[23,24] whereas others demonstrate less convincing improvements within surgical populations.[25] Debate on this subject continues, but the current rules set out by the Accreditation Council for Graduate Medical Education limit duty hours and abiding by these rules is part of current safety recommendations.

Electronic Order Entry

Additional system-improving recommendations include electronic order entry, which is primarily aimed at reducing medication errors, because these errors are the source of about 770,000 adverse events annually.[26,27] The highest-risk medications include insulin and heparin. In addition to computerizing order entry, there is much support for implementing standardized order sets for patients in multiple different settings.[28,29] Unfortunately, data regarding the effects of these interventions on the thoracic surgical population specifically are lacking, but again this is a current area of research.

Simulation

Simulation has been widely used in high-reliability organizations such as aviation and nuclear power plants but has been slow to be adopted by surgery. The hindrances are multifactorial and seem to be changing slowly. Simulation has been demonstrated to improve technical skills among surgical trainees and these skills are transferable to the operating room.[30] Beyond technical skills, simulation can be used to improve team performance, crisis management, and additional nonoperative technical skills. The impact of these of programs on errors and patient safety is a current area of research.

The impact of teaching surgical residents regarding patient safety has been the subject of many studies. Although some of the literature has suggested minimal impact or only an increase in time associated with operations performed by trainees, a recent study from the National Surgical Quality Improvement Project database reported a significant impact on not only operative times but also operative morbidity.[31] This is a growing concern for patients and their family members because these issues appear in the public domain. It is likely that continued highlighting of this area will push the incorporation of simulation further into the education of surgical trainees.

Telementoring

Telementoring has become a reality in concert with camera-driven procedures and the reliability of satellite transmission. In the review of several closed claims analysis of surgical errors, a common underlying theme supports lack of expertise as the significant source of error. Although it is in the early stages of development and incorporation, initial results show promise for the impact of telementoring for surgeons in the area of surgical expertise.[32,33]

SUMMARY

Constant vigilance examining the outcomes related to surgical interventions has led to a marked improvement in those outcomes during the past century. Surgeons work in an ever-increasing hazardous environment with more complex patient populations, risking injury to patients. Surgeons should embrace the cultural change necessary to prospectively study errors, learn from their occurrence, and implement change to prevent a future occurrence. They must be strong advocates for change within the system to help themselves and the other integral members of the surgical team trap errors before they reach patients. It is only through a conscious robust team approach to error identification and management that clinicians will slowly move toward safer health care for all.

REFERENCES

1. Kohn LT, Corrigan J, Donaldson MS, Institute of Medicine (US), Committee on Quality of Health Care in America. To err is human: building a safer health care system. Washington, DC: National Academies Press; 1999.
2. Gawande AA, Thomas EJ, Zinner MJ, et al. The incidence and nature of surgical adverse events in Colorado and Utah in 1992. Surgery 1999;126:66–75.
3. McGuire HH, Horsley JS, Salter DR, et al. Measuring and managing quality of surgery: statistical vs incidental approaches. Arch Surg 1992;127:733–8.

4. Donchin Y, Gopher D, Olin M, et al. A look into the nature and causes of human errors in the intensive care unit. Crit Care Med 1995;23(2):294–300.

5. Tinker JH, Dull DL, Caplan RA, et al. Role of monitoring devices in prevention of anesthetic mishaps: a closed claims analysis. Anesthesiology 1989;71:541–6.

6. Caplan RA, Posner KL, Ward RJ, et al. Adverse respiratory events in anesthesia: a closed claims analysis. Anesthesiology 1990;72:828–33.

7. Flin R, Maran N. Identifying and training non-technical skills for teams in acute medicine. Qual Saf Health Care 2004;13(Suppl 1):i80–4.

8. Healy AN, Undre S, Vincent C. Developing observational measures of performance in surgical teams. Qual Saf Health Care 2004;13:i33–40.

9. Wanzel KR, Jamieson CG, Bohnen JM. Complications on a general surgery service: incidence and reporting. Can J Surg 2000;43:113–7.

10. Cullen DJ, Bates DW, Small SD, et al. The incident reporting system does not detect adverse drug events: a problem for quality improve-ment. Jt Comm J Qual Improv 1995;21:541–8.

11. Lundy D, Laspina S, Kaplan H, et al. Seven hundred and fifty-nine (759) chances to learn: a 3-year pilot project to analyse transfusion-related near-miss events in the Republic of Ireland. Vox Sang 2007;92(3):233–41.

12. Helmreich RL. On error management: lessons from aviation. BMJ 2000;320:781–5.

13. Greenberg CC, Regenbogen SE, Studdert DM, et al. Patterns of communication breakdowns resulting in injury to surgical patients. J Am Coll Surg 2007; 204(4):533–40.

14. Van Eaton EG, Horvath KD, Lober WB, et al. A randomized, controlled trial evaluating the impact of a computerized rounding and sign-out system on continuity of care and resident work hours. J Am Coll Surg 2005;200(4):538–45.

15. Amato-Vealey EJ, Barba MP, Vealey RJ. Hand-off communication: a requisite for perioperative patient safety. AORN J 2008;88(5):763–70.

16. Nakayama DK, Lester SS, Rich DR, et al. Quality improvement and patient care checklists in intrahospital transfers involving pediatric surgery patients. J Pediatr Surg 2012;47(1):112–8.

17. Kim SW, Maturo S, Dwyer D, et al. Interdisciplinary development and implementation of communication checklist for postoperative management of pediatric airway patients. Otolaryngol Head Neck Surg 2012; 146(1):129–34.

18. Zavalkoff SR, Razack SI, Lavoie J, et al. Handover after pediatric heart surgery: a simple tool improves information exchange. Pediatr Crit Care Med 2011; 12(3):309–13.

19. Broom MA, Capek AL, Carachi P, et al. Critical phase distractions in anaesthesia and the sterile cockpit concept. Anaesthesia 2011;66(3):175–9.

20. Clarke JR, Johnston J, Blanco M, et al. Wrong-site surgery: can we prevent it? Adv Surg 2008;42:13–31.

21. Weiser TG, Haynes AB, Dziekan G, et al. Effect of a 19-item surgical safety checklist during urgent operations in a global patient population. Safe Surgery Saves Lives Investigators and Study Group. Ann Surg 2010;251(5):976–80.

22. de Vries EN, Eikens-Jansen MP, Hamersma AM, et al. Prevention of surgical malpractice claims by use of a surgical safety checklist. Ann Surg 2011; 253(3):624–8.

23. Lockley SW, Cronin JW, Evans EE, et al. Effect of reducing interns' weekly work hours on sleep and attentional failures. Harvard Work Hours, Health and Safety Group. N Engl J Med 2004;351(18): 1829–37.

24. Landrigan CP, Rothschild JM, Cronin JW, et al. Effect of reducing interns' work hours on serious medical errors in intensive care units. N Engl J Med 2004; 351(18):1838–48.

25. Helling TS, Kaswan S, Boccardo J, et al. The effect of resident duty hour restriction on trauma center outcomes in teaching hospitals in the state of Pennsylvania. J Trauma 2010;69(3):607–12.

26. Bates DW, Leape LL, Cullen DJ, et al. Effect of computerized physician order entry and a team intervention on prevention of serious medication errors. JAMA 1998;280(15):1311–6.

27. Lesar TS, Lomaestro BM, Pohl H. Medication-prescribing errors in a teaching hospital. A 9-year experience. Arch Intern Med 1997;157(14):1569–76.

28. Fleming NS, Ogola G, Ballard DJ. Implementing a standardized order set for community-acquired pneumonia: impact on mortality and cost. Jt Comm J Qual Patient Saf 2009;35(8):414–21.

29. Micek ST, Roubinian N, Heuring T, et al. Before-after study of a standardized hospital order set for the management of septic shock. Crit Care Med 2006; 34(11):2707–13.

30. Zendejas B, Cook DA, Bingener J, et al. Simulation-based mastery learning improves patient outcomes in laparoscopic inguinal hernia repair: a randomized controlled trial. Ann Surg 2011;254(3):502–9.

31. Advani V, Ahad S, Gonczy C, et al. Does resident involvement effect surgical times and complication rates during laparoscopic appendectomy for uncomplicated appendicitis? An analysis of 16,849 cases from the ACS-NSQIP. Am J Surg 2012; 203(3):347–51.

32. Okrainec A, Henao O, Azzie G. Telesimulation: an effective method for teaching the fundamentals of laparoscopic surgery in resource-restricted countries. Surg Endosc 2009;24(2):417–22.

33. Rosser JC, Wood M, Payne JH, et al. Telementoring. A practical option in surgical training. Surg Endosc 1997;11(8):852–5.

Patients' Satisfaction
Customer Relationship Management as a New Opportunity for Quality Improvement in Thoracic Surgery

Gaetano Rocco, MD, FRCSEd[a],*, Alessandro Brunelli, MD[b]

KEYWORDS

• Quality of care • Performance indicators • Patient satisfaction • Quality improvement

KEY POINTS

• Clinical and nonclinical indicators of performance are meant to provide the surgeon with tools to identify weaknesses to be improved.
• The World Health Organization's Performance Evaluation Systems (PES) represent a multidimensional approach to quality measurement based on several categories made of different indicators. Indicators for patient satisfaction may include overall perceived quality, accessibility, humanization and patient involvement, communication, and trust in health care providers.
• Patient satisfaction is included among nonclinical indicators of performance in thoracic surgery and is increasingly recognized as one of the outcome measures for delivered quality of care.

Worldwide, health systems are based on the concept of quality of care perceived by third party payers, but rarely by patients.[1] Undoubtedly, quality of care is a complex combination of the excellence in managed care and patients' perception of the best possible standards of care.[2,3] Whether cost-effectiveness is ever related to quality of care needs to be carefully ascertained.

Admittedly, patient-centered care, besides optimal clinical management, is based on (1) compassion, empathy, and responsiveness to needs, values, and expressed preferences; (2) coordination and integration; (3) information, communication, and education; (4) physical comfort; (5) emotional support, relieving fear and anxiety; and (6) involvement of family and friends.[4,5]

It seems a paradox that users of a service or, even more crudely, clients, are usually not listened to in evaluating a unit or a single surgeon's performances. Marketing makes this a fundamental rule of business: meet customers' expectations. Would one agree to buy a new car against his or her preferences? Could any retailing store function without a suitably located customer service facility?

THE PATIENT AS A CONSUMER

A patient becomes a consumer when he or she exercises the right to the best choice to diagnose and treat his or her medical condition based on the available information and in his or her best interest.[6] The patient-consumer role is being redefined at different socioeconomic environments at different latitudes regardless of the available provision of care.[7,8] As an example, in a socialized medicine model, to diagnose and treat any medical condition, patients may have the option of private practice but also of institutions with a similar spectrum of services but away from regional facilities. The only difference lies in the coverage of medical expenses, which, in the latter circumstance, is still provided by social

a Division of Thoracic Surgery, Department of Thoracic Surgery and Oncology, National Cancer Institute, Pascale Foundation, Via Mariano Semmola 81 80131 Naples, Italy; b Division of Thoracic Surgery, Ospedali Riuniti, Via Conca 71, Torrette, Ancona, Italy
* Corresponding author.
E-mail address: Gaetano.Rocco@btopenworld.com

Thorac Surg Clin 22 (2012) 551–555
http://dx.doi.org/10.1016/j.thorsurg.2012.07.009
1547-4127/12/$ – see front matter © 2012 Elsevier Inc. All rights reserved.

welfare. Moreover, besides freedom of choice, patients/consumers request more information, equitable access to health care, prompt attention, respect, and quality of amenities.[7,8]

THE PATIENT/CUSTOMER'S SATISFACTION

Patient's satisfaction is a difficult concept to fully define, as it consists of a multifactorial, subjective judgment often related with an inverse ratio to the level of knowledge of the service the patient is offered.[9] Indeed, if patients have minimal knowledge and expectations of service quality, the chance of recording higher satisfaction is significant. Conversely, the reverse can be true when highly educated patients may not find enough quality regardless of outstanding service features. Hence, dissatisfaction and satisfaction may be generated each from different socioeconomic and cultural factors.[9] As a consequence, the jury is still out whether, as it is, patient satisfaction should be used as a surrogate of the overall quality of service.[9]

MEASURING PATIENT SATISFACTION

In recent years, with the increasing interest in patient satisfaction, it became clear that an objective measurement of this nonclinical parameter had to be introduced.[10] The basic tenet supporting this need is that satisfied patients do participate to a greater and better extent in their process of care.[11] In other words, they become better consumers. However, objective measurements are often structured according to the provider's perspective rather than the patient's.[1] The World Health Organization has included patient perspectives, satisfaction, or patient centeredness among the targets to be evaluated in the so-called Performance Evaluation Systems or PES.[12] PES represent a multidimensional approach to quality measurement based on several categories made of different indicators.[13] Indicators for patient satisfaction may include, among others, overall perceived quality, accessibility, humanization and patient involvement, communication, and trust in health care providers. Surveys are usually distributed among patients and data are entered into mathematical models to quantify the dimension "patient satisfaction."[14]

PATIENT SATISFACTION IN GENERAL THORACIC SURGERY

Patient satisfaction is included among nonclinical indicators of performance in thoracic surgery and is increasingly recognized as one of the outcome measures of the delivered quality of care.[15] Barlési and colleagues[16] analyzed patient satisfaction

following major pulmonary resections in an effort to verify a possible link between patient satisfaction and quality of care. Global staff and structure mean patient satisfaction was 78% ($\pm$13% SD) and 69% ($\pm$13%), respectively. Although overall quality of surgical care was rated 88%, a correlation with patient satisfaction was not demonstrated.[16] In 2009, Rocco and colleagues published on the principles of PES and in particular on patient satisfaction in thoracic surgery as one item of the multidimensional approach to quality measurement.[10] An itemized questionnaire containing 37 multiple-choice questions was distributed among 79 patients undergoing thoracic surgical procedures.[10] The questions addressed 5 categories of patient experience during hospitalization: perceived quality of facilities, quality and clarity of the provided information, quality of the relationship with surgeons and nurses, quality of the received care, and overall patient satisfaction.[10] To explore these categories, 29 different indicators of the hospitalization were addressed in the 37 questions, each graded on a 1 to 6 scale with 6 attributed to the highest perceived quality.[10] In addition, cluster analysis was used to stratify responses by socioeconomic classes according to the procedure of automatic classification (Ward's method).[10] Indeed, with cluster analysis, Rocco and colleagues[10] were able to classify consumers into 4 groups, homogeneous within each group as to age, geographic origin, level of education, and current occupation and maximize the differences of perceived quality among these groups. Partial least squares regression model was used to correlate indicators to categories of perceived quality and patient satisfaction (**Fig. 1**).[10] Overall, a 92% satisfaction rate was observed with highest perceived quality among female patients from the suburban areas of Naples.[10] In addition, the analysis demonstrated that waiting times for radiological procedures, quality of meals, and duration of visiting hours were the issues generating dissatisfaction (**Fig. 2**).[10] It appears obvious that such an evaluation enables the surgeon/administrator to identify potential weaknesses in the provision of care and accordingly allocate human and technical resources.[10]

Recently, patient satisfaction was compared in 2 thoracic surgical centers in Italy by distributing the EORTC-InPatSat32 module to 280 consecutive patients undergoing thoracic surgical procedures during a 2-year period.[17] Interestingly, differences in the doctors-related indicators (ie, technical and interpersonal skills, physician availability, and provision of information) were the only determinants of higher perceived quality from patients of one unit.[17] Multivariable regression with bootstrap

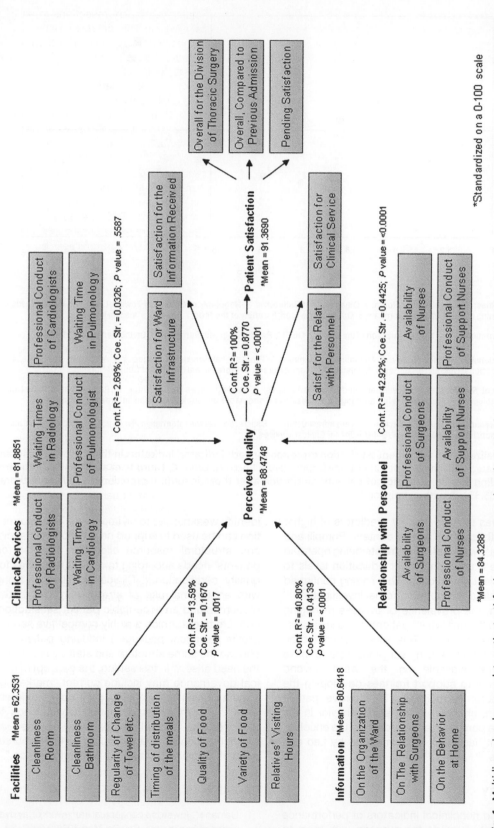

Fig. 1. Multidimensional approach to patient satisfaction measurement based on several categories made of different indicators exploring perceived quality of facilities, delivery of information, clinical services, and relationship with personnel. The overall perceived quality was significantly correlated to patient satisfaction. (*From* Rocco G, Lauro C, Lauro N, et al. Partial least squares path modeling for the evaluation of patients' satisfaction after thoracic surgical procedures. Eur J Cardiothorac Surg 2009;35:353–7; with permission.)

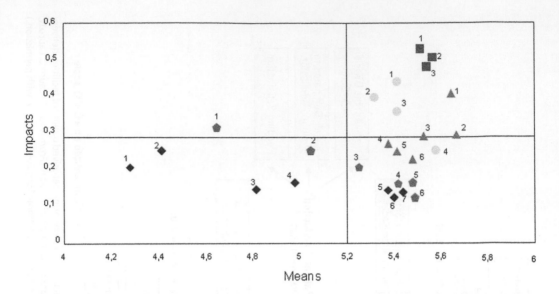

Facilities: 1. Cleanliness of Room; 2. Cleanliness of Bathrooms; 3. Regularity of Change of Towels, Linen and Bed Spreads; 4. Timing of distribution of the meals; 5. Quality of the food; 6.Variety of the food; 7. Relatives' visiting hours.

Information: 1. On the Organization of the Ward; 2. On The Relationship with Surgeons; 3. On the Behavior at Home.

Relationship with Personnel: 1. Availability of Surgeons; 2. Professional Conduct of Surgeons; 3. Availability of Nurses; 4. Professional Conduct of Nurses; 5. Availability of Support Nurses; 6. Professional Conduct of Support Nurses.

Clinical Services: 1. Professional Conduct of Radiologists; 2. Waiting Times in Radiology; 3. Professional Conduct of Cardiologists; 4. Waiting Time in Cardiology; 5. Professional Conduct of Pulmonologist; 6. Waiting Time in Pulmonology.

Perceived Quality: 1. Satisfaction for Ward Infrastructure; 2. Satisfaction for the Information Received; 3. Satisfaction for the Relationship with Personnel; 4. Satisfaction for Clinical Services.

Fig. 2. Visualization of the patient satisfaction expressed for each indicator; indicators in the left lower quadrant were correlated with the lowest patient satisfaction. (*From* Rocco G, Lauro C, Lauro N, et al. Partial least squares path modeling for the evaluation of patients' satisfaction after thoracic surgical procedures. Eur J Cardiothorac Surg 2009;35:353–7; with permission.)

analysis was used to identify predictors of higher patient satisfaction.[17] In this context, Pompili and colleagues[17] were able to correlate being operated in 1 of the 2 units and lower education levels to higher patient satisfaction. This finding confirmed what was already reported by other investigators.[16] In addition, the prevalence of trainees managing the ward in the unit where patients were less satisfied was noteworthy.[17] This aspect prompted an alteration of the attending surgeons' rota to make them more available on the ward beyond usual rounds to support trainees developing the patient-doctor relationship. To improve patient satisfaction, changes in the staff behavior in the setting of a personalized approach to the oncological patient has been recommended by Leo and colleagues.[18]

identify weaknesses to be improved. This information can be used to support negotiation of financial and structural resource allocation focused on patients' needs according to current requisites for quality certification.[19] Clinical excellence, along with an optimal use of strategically distributed resources and an acceptable patient satisfaction, concurs to determine a highly competitive service profile ("surgical package") inducing patients to choose the same structure and staff again, should the need arise.[20] In this setting, the concept of clinical governance may include current "marketing" criteria, which are applied to compare different units.[21] Patient satisfaction rightfully belongs to these criteria and will increasingly be used as a benchmarking indicator for third party reimbursement strategies such as "pay per performance."[22]

SUMMARY

Clinical and nonclinical indicators of performance are meant to provide the surgeon with tools to

REFERENCES

1. Calnan M. Towards a conceptual framework of lay evaluation of health care. Soc Sci Med 1988;27:927–33.

2. The World Health Report 2000. Health Systems: improving performance. Geneva (Switzerland): World Health Organization; 2000.

3. Donabedian A. Quality assessment and assurance: unity of purpose, diversity of means. Inquiry 1988; 25:173–92.

4. Goodrich J, Cornwell J. Seeing the person in the patient. The Point of Care review paper. London: The King's Fund; 2008. p. 6–17.

5. Institute of Medicine. Crossing the quality chasm: a new health system for the 21st century. Washington, DC: National Academy Press; 2001.

6. Shackley P, Ryan M. What is the role of the consumer in health care? J Soc Policy 1994;23:517–41.

7. Coulter A, Jenkinson J. European patients' views on the responsiveness of health systems and healthcare providers. Eur J Public Health 2005;15:355–60.

8. Hudak PL, McKeever P, Wright JG. The metaphor of patient as customers: implication for measuring satisfaction. J Clin Epidemiol 2003;56:103–8.

9. Avis M, Bond M, Arthur A. Satisfying solutions? A review of some unresolved issues in the measurement of patient satisfaction. J Adv Nurs 1995;22: 316–22.

10. Rocco G, Lauro C, Lauro N, et al. Partial least squares path modelling for the evaluation of patients' satisfaction after thoracic surgical procedures. Eur J Cardiothorac Surg 2009;35:353–7.

11. Guldvog B. Can patient satisfaction improve health among patients with angina pectoris? Int J Qual Health Care 1999;11:233–40.

12. Arah OA, Klazinga NS, Delnoij DM, et al. Conceptual frameworks for health systems performance: a quest for effectiveness, quality, and improvement. Int J Qual Health Care 2003;15:377–98.

13. Hekkert KD, Cihangir S, Kleefstra SM, et al. Patient satisfaction revisited: a multilevel approach. Soc Sci Med 2009;69:68–75.

14. González N, Quintana JM, Bilbao A, et al. Development and validation of an in-patient satisfaction questionnaire. Int J Qual Health Care 2005;17:465–72.

15. Brunelli A, Rocco G. Clinical and nonclinical indicators of performance in thoracic surgery. Thorac Surg Clin 2007;17:369–77.

16. Barlési F, Boyer L, Doddoli C, et al. The place of patient satisfaction in quality assessment of lung cancer thoracic surgery. Chest 2005;128:3475–81.

17. Pompili C, Brunelli A, Rocco G, et al. Patient satisfaction after pulmonary resection for lung cancer: a multicenter comparative analysis. Respiration, in press.

18. Leo F, Radice D, Didier F, et al. Does a personalized approach improve patient satisfaction in thoracic oncology? Am J Manag Care 2009;15:361–7.

19. Veillard J, Champagne F, Klazinga N, et al. A performance assessment framework for hospitals: the WHO regional office for Europe PATH project. Int J Qual Health Care 2005;17:487–96.

20. Seghieri C, Sandoval GA, Brown AD, et al. Where to focus efforts to improve overall ratings of care and willingness to return: the case of Tuscan emergency departments. Acad Emerg Med 2009;16:136–44.

21. Brunelli A, Rocco G. The comparison of performance between thoracic surgical units. Thorac Surg Clin 2007;17:413–24.

22. Varela G. Pay for performance in thoracic surgery. Thorac Surg Clin 2007;17:431–5.

Index

Thorac Surg Clin 22 (2012) 557–560
http://dx.doi.org/10.1016/S1547-4127(12)00066-7
1547-4127/12/$ – see front matter © 2012 Elsevier Inc. All rights reserved.

United States Postal Service

Statement of Ownership, Management, and Circulation
(All Periodicals Publications Except Requestor Publications)

1. Publication Title	2. Publication Number	3. Filing Date
Thoracic Surgery Clinics	0 1 3 - 1 2 6	9/14/12

4. Issue Frequency	5. Number of Issues Published Annually	6. Annual Subscription Price
Feb, May, Aug, Nov	4	$322.00

7. Complete Mailing Address of Known Office of Publication (Not printer) (Street, city, county, state, and ZIP+4®)

Elsevier Inc.
360 Park Avenue South
New York, NY 10010-1710

Contact Person
Stephen R. Bushing

Telephone (Include area code)
215-239-3688

8. Complete Mailing Address of Headquarters or General Business Office of Publisher (Not printer)

Elsevier Inc., 360 Park Avenue South, New York, NY 10010-1710

9. Full Names and Complete Mailing Addresses of Publisher, Editor, and Managing Editor (Do not leave blank)

Publisher (Name and complete mailing address)

Kim Murphy, Elsevier, Inc., 1600 John F. Kennedy Blvd. Suite 1800, Philadelphia, PA 19103-2899

Editor (Name and complete mailing address)

Barbara Cohen-Kligerman, Elsevier, Inc., 1600 John F. Kennedy Blvd. Suite 1800, Philadelphia, PA 19103-2899

Managing Editor (Name and complete mailing address)

Barbara Cohen-Kligerman, Elsevier, Inc., 1600 John F. Kennedy Blvd. Suite 1800, Philadelphia, PA 19103-2899

10. Owner (Do not leave blank. If the publication is owned by a corporation, give the name and address of the corporation immediately followed by the names and addresses of all stockholders owning or holding 1 percent or more of the total amount of stock. If not owned by a corporation, give the names and addresses of the individual owners. If owned by a partnership or other unincorporated firm, give its name and address as well as those of each individual owner. If the publication is published by a nonprofit organization, give its name and address.)

Full Name	Complete Mailing Address
Wholly owned subsidiary of	1600 John F. Kennedy Blvd., Ste. 1800
Reed/Elsevier, US holdings	Philadelphia, PA 19103-2899

11. Known Bondholders, Mortgagees, and Other Security Holders Owning or Holding 1 Percent or More of Total Amount of Bonds, Mortgages, or Other Securities. If none, check box ☐ None

Full Name	Complete Mailing Address
N/A	

12. Tax Status (For completion by nonprofit organizations authorized to mail at nonprofit rates) (Check one)
The purpose, function, and nonprofit status of this organization and the exempt status for federal income tax purposes:
☐ Has Not Changed During Preceding 12 Months
☐ Has Changed During Preceding 12 Months (Publisher must submit explanation of change with this statement)

PS Form 3526, September 2007 (Page 1 of 3 (Instructions Page 3)) PSN 7530-01-000-9931 PRIVACY NOTICE: See our Privacy policy in www.usps.com

---

13. Publication Title	14. Issue Date for Circulation Data Below
Thoracic Surgery Clinics	August 2012

15. Extent and Nature of Circulation		Average No. Copies Each Issue During Preceding 12 Months	No. Copies of Single Issue Published Nearest to Filing Date
a. Total Number of Copies (Net press run)		913	726
b. Paid Circulation (By Mail and Outside the Mail)	(1) Mailed Outside-County Paid Subscriptions Stated on PS Form 3541. (Include paid distribution above nominal rate, advertiser's proof copies, and exchange copies)	468	437
	(2) Mailed In-County Paid Subscriptions Stated on PS Form 3541 (Include paid distribution above nominal rate, advertiser's proof copies, and exchange copies)		
	(3) Paid Distribution Outside the Mails Including Sales Through Dealers and Carriers, Street Vendors, Counter Sales, and Other Paid Distribution Outside USPS®	161	181
	(4) Paid Distribution by Other Classes Mailed Through the USPS (e.g. First-Class Mail®)		
c. Total Paid Distribution (Sum of 15b (1), (2), (3), and (4))	▲	629	618
d. Free or Nominal Rate Distribution (By Mail and Outside the Mail)	(1) Free or Nominal Rate Outside-County Copies Included on PS Form 3541	52	54
	(2) Free or Nominal Rate In-County Copies Included on PS Form 3541		
	(3) Free or Nominal Rate Copies Mailed at Other Classes Through the USPS (e.g. First-Class Mail)		
	(4) Free or Nominal Rate Distribution Outside the Mail (Carriers or other means)		
e. Total Free or Nominal Rate Distribution (Sum of 15d (1), (2), (3) and (4))	▲	52	54
f. Total Distribution (Sum of 15c and 15e)		681	672
g. Copies not Distributed (See instructions to publishers #4 (page #3))	▲	232	54
h. Total (Sum of 15f and g)	▲	913	726
i. Percent Paid (15c divided by 15f times 100)		92.36%	91.96%

16. Publication of Statement of Ownership

☐ If the publication is a general publication, publication of this statement is required. Will be printed in the November 2012 issue of this publication. ☐ Publication not required

17. Signature and Title of Editor, Publisher, Business Manager, or Owner	Date
[signature] Stephen R. Bushing –Inventory/Distribution Coordinator	September 14, 2012

I certify that all information furnished on this form is true and complete. I understand that anyone who furnishes false or misleading information on this form or who omits material or information requested on the form may be subject to criminal sanctions (including fines and imprisonment) and/or civil sanctions (including civil penalties).

PS Form 3526, September 2007 (Page 2 of 3)

Moving?

Make sure your subscription moves with you!

To notify us of your new address, find your **Clinics Account Number** (located on your mailing label above your name), and contact customer service at:

Email: journalscustomerservice-usa@elsevier.com

800-654-2452 (subscribers in the U.S. & Canada)
314-447-8871 (subscribers outside of the U.S. & Canada)

Fax number: 314-447-8029

Elsevier Health Sciences Division
Subscription Customer Service
3251 Riverport Lane
Maryland Heights, MO 63043

*To ensure uninterrupted delivery of your subscription, please notify us at least 4 weeks in advance of move.

Printed and bound by CPI Group (UK) Ltd, Croydon, CR0 4YY

03/10/2024

01040354-0004